Praise for *Hairlooms*

"Entertaining and educational, *Hairlooms* is a wonderful tool for self-correction and self-discovery."

—Felicia Leatherwood,
natural hair celebrity stylist

"*Hairlooms* provides a beautiful reflection of how the natural hair journey evolves into inner transformation. Michele gives you the tools for your own self-reflection and empowers you to tell your own story!"

—Mae aka Natural Chica,
natural hair and lifestyle blogger

"As someone who has worked to empower and educate people to accept their natural hair for the past eighteen years, I loved *Hairlooms!* It was an inspiring reminder of the power that each of us has within us to embrace our natural beauty. Through Michele's story and the stories of some of the top influencers in the natural hair world, she provides a powerful read that helps readers navigate the process of loving their hair and beauty."

—Michelle Breyer,
cofounder, head of business development,
TextureMedia LLC, which includes
NaturallyCurly, CurlyNikki, and CurlMart

"You will not leave this book without dancing! *Hairlooms* is a healing party and perfect for the Black woman's journey toward self-love."

—Joiya Cloud,
Fros & Beaus, Instagram platform

"*Hairlooms* carefully combs through every emotion that African-American women feel about hair and beauty. This book is truly inspirational, no matter where you are in your hair journey. Thank you, Michele, for giving voice to issues that African-American women are facing."

—Christina Miracle Bailey,
District of Columbia Library Association Past President

"As a new father, *Hairlooms* is so necessary. We want our little girl to love and enjoy her hair in all of its natural beauty. It's one thing to want to try different styles; it's another thing to hate the natural hair you were born with! *Hairlooms* is an awesome tool to plant self-love in a little girl's heart during the earliest phases of her life."

—La Guardia Cross,
"New Father Chronicles" YouTube sensation

"Wow! Reading *Hairlooms* was soothing and familiar, like the best scalp massage you've ever had . . . the one where the shampoo girl really *gets in there* and scrubs away a week of worries. Michele's story is one of vulnerability, discovery, and self-acceptance detangled with words before our eyes. It's interwoven with stories of other Black women sharing their own hair journey, pains, revelations, and redemptions. I found myself pulled in by her writing and sliding effortlessly through each chapter like a wide-toothed comb through conditioner-covered tresses. *Hairlooms* is a brave and beautiful gift to readers who are ready to affirm their own beauty, inside and out."

—Roshini Cope,
Galamazini, beauty, health, and wellness blogger/vlogger

"*Hairlooms* is a very inspiring and fascinating book. I reside in Nigeria, and the natural hair community is growing steadily, but there is still more work to be done. Unfortunately, so many Nigerian women believe that people who wear their hair natural are too poor to get relaxers. *Hairlooms* is a book African-American mothers, fathers, and even youth must read. Some of these hair stories should even be read to little girls; each one will help them accept their unique physical qualities and get inspired!"

—The Curly Belle,
natural hair blogger

HAIRLOOMS

The Untangled Truth About
Loving Your Natural Hair and Beauty

MICHELE TAPP ROSEMAN

158
R

Health Communications, Inc.
Deerfield Beach, Florida

www.hcibooks.com

Library of Congress Cataloging-in-Publication Data
is available through the Library of Congress

© 2017 Michele Tapp Roseman

ISBN-13: 978-07573-1967-9 (Paperback)
ISBN-10: 07573-1967-X (Paperback)
ISBN-13: 978-07573-1968-6 (ePub)
ISBN-10: 07573-1968-8 (ePub)

HCI, its logos, and marks are trademarks of Health Communications, Inc.

Publisher: Health Communications, Inc.
    3201 S.W. 15th Street
    Deerfield Beach, FL 33442–8190

Cover design by Andrea Perrine Brower
Interior design and formatting by Lawna Patterson Oldfield

I dedicate *Hairlooms* to my "natural" sister, Sheila.
Thank you for teaching me how to handle my history,
my healing, and—most of all—my hair.

I love you.

Contents

Acknowledgments

Before all others, thank you **God** for the September "aha" moment that set the *Hairlooms* book project in motion. Your ability to extract beauty and purpose from my most painful moments leaves me speechless. The way in which you connect the dots between people, space, and time is simply amazing and always unmatched.

To my husband and "sole" mate Kyle: You've been there to see my mistakenly bright yellow-dyed hair, the transition from permed to natural hair, several twist-out fails, and the long journey to love myself! You never judged. You never laughed. You never criticized. You never left. Your presence, silence, and gentle prodding have been just what I have needed to make it through. Who would have thought this book project would take more than six years? We didn't, but I made it through because you were with me every step of the way. You are a great man. I honor, respect, and love you.

Mother and Daddy: Thank you for selflessly giving me the best parts of yourselves. Every ounce of creativity and freedom to express comes from what I have received from you. I'm so glad you never squelched my flame. Whether I was playing the piano or turning a jewelry box into a makeshift cash register, you accepted my gifts and gave me the wings and wind I needed to fly.

Mom and Dad Roseman, and Raven and Marcus: For the countless times you checked on the book during our road trips and Cracker Barrel stops—thank you. Since day one, you've always cheered me on, and I appreciate your support during the *Hairlooms* journey. My project never went unnoticed by you. Your love never goes unnoticed by me.

Olivia Savannah Logan, your transcription and research skills were unforgettable. I appreciate you for always sending the unexpected when I least expected it but needed it the most. Thanks for being more than my cousin; thank you for being my friend.

Cheryl Black, Esq: Who would have thought that our introduction as twenty-somethings would lead us to work together almost twenty years later? Your wisdom has been a complete godsend. I'll never forget your challenge to "put blood on the pages." Most of all, I'll never forget your friendship. Thank you.

I think it's safe to say that most literary agents find the client once the story has been written. **Claudia Menza**, I'm grateful that you saw the *Hairlooms* vision while it was still in the making. Your sound literary insights and expertise have provided the gentle steering I needed to stay on course and bring my "craft" safely to shore. From one curly woman to another, I appreciate you—many thanks!

To the **HCI Books team**, I appreciate the respect, care, and professionalism with which you have handled my vision—thank you.

To every **contributor**, thank you for granting me the privilege of telling your story. We seldom allow outsiders into our space. You, however, believed in the *Hairlooms* project and made room for me when you could have easily closed the door. As a body of contributors, your tenacity to remain vulnerable and transparent has been a gift. I can't wait for readers to unwrap a section of your lives—as I have.

Preface

> *"There is no serendipity . . . only Divinity."*
>
> —Michele Tapp Roseman

I'll never forget Thursday, September 16, 2010.

Expectant people scurried from room to room in hopes of arriving right on time for the impending birth. The atmosphere was electric. There were no instrument-carrying obstetricians or mask-clad midwives on hand. I do, however, recall seeing some stylish Ann Taylor and St. John Knit suits. There was a birth that day, but I was *not* in a maternity ward. This was the day I conceived the idea for *Hairlooms* at the Walter E. Washington Convention Center in Washington, D.C.!

I was wearing a pink boucle skirt suit and brushed gold ballerina slippers. I know that pumps would have been a better complement to my suit, but smart women know that the Walter E. Washington Convention Center's 700,000-plus feet of exhibit space is *not* the place for stilettos. I had just spent this fall day attending the Congressional Black Caucus Foundation's (CBCF) Annual Legislative Conference events. My bunions were grateful for my "sole" choice and held up quite well during my trek to become informed—and occasionally grab vendor freebies along the way.

While I wasn't scheduled to speak during any CBCF brain trusts or to moderate panel discussions, I nevertheless felt like a bit of a celebrity. From the corner of my mind's eye, I started noticing that wherever I went, Black women would stop me to talk about my hair. The joy of these encounters didn't mask the fact that I still felt awkward about wearing my curly Afro. The last thing I wanted to do was chat it up with complete strangers about my hair. I knew I looked presentable but didn't feel ready for the New York Fashion Week runway yet. We all know what that discomfort is like. It's the feeling you get right before you rock your "trending" purple lipstick and hope you don't look like you ate a tub full of blueberries. It's the uneasiness you get before squeezing into your "prayer pants"—the pants we pray don't pop a button or rip at the seams because they are a size too small.

"How long have you been natural?" someone asked.

I sheepishly replied, "I guess about two years. I didn't really keep track. I just remember it was around my birthday."

Another stranger asked, "What did you use to get your hair like that?"

I mustered a lackluster, but true, response. "I started trying different products and found something that worked for me." Product failure was a pain point for most women I met.

"That hair custard didn't curl my hair," one stranger complained.

I encouraged her to "find a product that works for you and go with that." After dodging a few more questions and completing my eight-hour convention center marathon, I was pooped. *Whew!* What a whirlwind day.

As I left the convention center, I mentally calculated the many mini conversations I'd had about my hair. This led to other memories of random women who excitedly asked me about my hair in the New York City Port Authority bus terminal. The natural hair styling tips I rushed to suggest before boarding a Maryland-bound bus made them smile. I recalled yet another encounter with a forlorn lady at a beauty supply store's checkout counter. She shared the heartbreak of a receding hairline and damaged hair follicles. More aware than ever, the obviously balding Black woman linked her hair woes to chemical treatments and openly struggled to live her present life without her former companion. Most of these conversations flowed with the ease of well-conditioned hair slipping through a wide-toothed comb. Although we were strangers at first, our talks about the "big chop" and two-strand twists made us "fro friends" within moments. Now, I don't want to paint an unrealistic picture of my encounters. It's not like I attracted thousands of women. I will say, though, that the regularity with which I was approached even piqued my husband Kyle's curiosity. He jokingly said I must be wearing an invisible "Ask Me About My Hair" neon sign.

Stunned by this mixture of memories, I had my epiphany after leaving the convention center and walking to my parked car. It was then that I was inspired to pen *Hairlooms*. At a very basic level, I was encouraged to tell people about my path toward self-acceptance, and a component of this, of course, included talking about accepting my hair. On a deeper level, I really knew this was not just about me and my personal journey—other women likely had a story to tell—so I decided to conduct interviews about the subject, and I soon realized my inklings were spot on. The thirty-two *Hairlooms'* interviewees—hailing from Alabama to Australia—confirmed my inner nudging and shared poignant hair experiences for this book. These extraordinary women and men gifted me with rich stories that unfolded at the intersection where hair and heart matters collide. Their personal insights helped me see what I sensed: "combing through" hair issues is a necessary gateway to achieving greater levels of self-acceptance.

The ancient Chinese philosopher Lao Tzu said, "A journey of a thousand miles must begin with a single step." After figuratively stepping across emotional terrain for five years (or 1,825 days), I felt that I had definitely been on a journey! Since taking my first step to write *Hairlooms* in September 2010, I've navigated through a lot of seasons. Admittedly, I don't remember everything else that happened that month. I'm not sure how much I weighed at the beginning of the month. I don't recall what lipstick I wore at the end of the month, but one thing's for sure:

On September 16, 2010, I was definitely having a "good hair day."

Introduction

Here's a riddle: What is strong enough to make some women refuse to exercise or get wet, yet weak enough to break from the ravages of chemotherapy and autoimmune disease? A woman's body is covered with 100,000 of them, and she recycles 100 of them daily.

Its flow and sway rivals the lushness of a tropical paradise. The wise admire it from afar and touch it only by invitation. Tied down at night, in the morning it rises up again like a phoenix, and can flourish despite intense heat and harsh chemicals. Released by some to explore robust expression, it's been known to cause a double take. From project stoops to penthouse steps, "sheroes" of the ages have dared to control, curl, and color it. Reducing some women to tears when cut, one inch of "new growth" can make them strut with peacock pride.

Do you know what it is? Undeniably complex. Unabashedly beautiful. Some call it "glory." It is your hair.

I wrote *Hairlooms: The Untangled Truth About Loving Your Natural Hair and Beauty* to help Black women—and people connected to us—identify and explore issues that may keep Black women from completely embracing our natural hair and inherent beauty. At some level, all of us know that hair issues dangle beyond texture and length.

1

Even today, at this point in history, we have pleasant and painful memories that are clear indicators that the validity of our beauty seems to rest on the type, length, and number of strands that adorn our heads.

Dating back to early memories, many of us realized that our hair could elicit praise or criticism. Some of us know the prestige of being favored because our manageable locks hugged our shoulders and responded like well-behaved children. Pressed hair that refused to unwind in the presence of summer's sweltering heat may still be a familiar sweet spot in our minds. Others can't forget how quickly our confidence evaporated beneath the scorch of an elder's biting comments about our tightly coiled locks.

Afro-textured hair has also faced scrutiny in many public arenas. Dialogue about the impact of the United States military's hairstyle ban—on Black female soldiers—caused an about-face on policy within the United States Army, United States Navy, and United States Air Force. On August 13, 2014, then United States Secretary of Defense, Chuck Hagel, overruled the armed forces' 239-year grooming code that restricted Black women's hairstyles.[1] This move was followed by the December 2015 decision that the United States Marines would modify its uniform policy.[2] In light of allegations of racial insensitivity, female Marines are now allowed to wear "locs" in their hair while in uniform.

In June 2014, NBC Today anchor Tamron Hall's big "natural curl" hair reveal created a stir in national and local media.[3] Sparks of controversy flew nationally as young Vanessa VanDyke faced bullying and suspension for wearing her natural, Afro-textured hair to school in 2013.[4] On the entertainment front, comedian Sheryl Underwood's August 2013 references to Black hair being "nasty" and "nappy" during a re-broadcast of *The Talk* did not go unnoticed.[5] The rapid-fire tweet-back in the Twittersphere precipitated her quick-response apology in September 2013, during Steve Harvey's nationally syndicated radio show. The topic of Black women's natural hair and obesity was even a discussion topic on Katie Couric's talk show, *Katie*.[6]

I have personally witnessed how the perceived texture of Black women's hair has even been fodder for discussion about animals. I love to crochet and wanted to get a close-up look at genuine alpaca fiber, so I went on a tour of an alpaca farm that was connected to a yarn shop near my house in the spring of 2016. During the tour, one of the breeders casually told our group of visitors—a racially mixed group—that the creamy white alpaca fleece is always preferred to the chocolaty brown alpaca fleece. The breeder matter-of-factly validated this claim by making a comparison between the "obvious" desirability of a White woman's hair texture versus a Black woman's hair texture. I was shocked, but it happened so quickly and was so outlandish that I didn't even think to respond.

This audacious comparison underscores the often-predictable public impressions about our Afro-textured, curly hair. Yale University's "First Impressions and Hair Impressions" study was conducted to explore whether observers determine a person's character traits solely by virtue of their hairstyles.[7] The introduction stated:

> As children, we were told not to judge a book by its cover, that things are not always what they seem, that appearances are beguiling, and that all that glitters is not gold. As adults, however, we cannot seem to help ourselves. A quick glance of someone is often enough to form a distinct first impression.

Based on hairstyles, study participants were asked to judge whether models possessed several social attributes. Respondents were asked to determine—by sight—whether the models were intelligent, sexy, or poor. Overwhelmingly, empirical data from this study revealed that the models with long, blond, and straight hair were perceived as beautiful and smart.

After reflecting on these findings and personal experiences, I could not help but wonder what these "first impressions" mean for women like us. We represent the women who—more often than not—don't have long, blond, straight hair. Genetic influences naturally place the majority of Black women in the "undesirable" category and leave the masses thinking we are dumb, unattractive, and poor.

While these insights have been the grounds for robust private and public discussions about our hair and beauty, the biggest question in my mind has been: *How do I move past the point of not completely accepting what I see in the mirror?*

For those of us who want to have a better grasp of our inherent beauty, we need to draw insights from another side of the natural hair and beauty discussion. Emotions definitely have a place in self-acceptance, but progress without hard data is just emotion. Personal experiences have taught me that the power needed for a genuine self-embrace is born of a mixture of feelings and fact. To this point, *Hairlooms* acknowledges some questions that may be absent from our natural-hair discussions. The first question is: *Why is it so difficult for Black women to embrace their hair and beauty?* The second question is: *How can Black women overcome the multi-layered challenge of embracing their natural hair and beauty?*

If we do the work and begin unearthing some personal truths, we will be poised to more clearly understand the genesis of any personal discomfort surrounding this topic. Moreover, we won't get tangled at pain points, but we will have a better understanding of how to make intentional, sustainable forward movement for ourselves. I know we are a lot of things to many people. I am a wife. You are a mother. We are money-makers and the shoulders upon which friends have cried. Before we ever assumed any of these titles, I was simply *me* and you were simply *you*.

I wrote *Hairlooms* for me, and I wrote it for you. After you read it, you will be in a position to:

- Understand why you—and other Black women—may have difficulty accepting your hair and beauty;
- Identify, discover, and overcome the internal roadblocks that hinder some Black women from accepting themselves; and
- Develop a deeper appreciation for your inner and outer beauty.

While *Hairlooms* addresses issues that directly impact Black women, I intentionally wanted to open the door for other groups who have questions about, or aren't familiar with, the array of challenges many of us face. Recent spikes in interracial marriages and transracial adoptions signal the need for answers to basic questions they may have, such as, "How do I handle a child's hair that is not like my own?" This book also bridges the information gap for men who are connected with us. We all know that touching our hair at the wrong time or making a snide remark about our looks can be grounds for a civil war. In their defense, a lot of times, the men in our worlds—Black and White—are honestly not aware of the deep-rooted self-acceptance issues we carry about our hair and beauty. Left unchecked, we may find ourselves in relationships with emotional snarls and knots that are hard to undo.

What to Expect

For starters, this book is really centered on my timeless truth: words shape worth. Accordingly, it comes as no surprise that the rise and fall of many Black women's self-perceptions of their hair and beauty is drawn from words. For the sake of this book, I refer to these identity-defining words with my self-created term, "hairlooms." An obvious play on the word *heirlooms*, this term refers to words about Black women's hair and beauty that are deemed worthy to pass along.

We all know that heirlooms are objects of great value that are handed down through several generations. Granddaddy's jewel-encrusted crucifix, Great-Great Auntie's secret family cheese biscuit recipes, and Great-Great-Great Grandmother's patchwork quilt make our hearts swell with pride and curl our lips with laughter. Heirlooms assure us that family torches will remain brightly lit in the wake of future millennia.

Tangible items are not the only markers of history. Code words about our hair may also create patterns that inevitably punctuate our family lines. Big Mama compared your mother's hair to *steel wool*. Your mother rolled her eyes and complained that your *nappy head* was too hard to comb. Now you refuse to compliment your niece until she gets a *fresh perm*. No doubt these phrases have been passed along generationally. Alternatively, "hairlooms" have been passed along generationally in private and public settings. These words, looks, and gestures have shaped our attraction or repulsion to certain types of hair and physical features.

Based on the power of words, *Hairlooms* is chock-full of word pictures and stories about this thought-provoking topic. In each chapter, you will find the following:

MY STORY

Every chapter paints a picture of the steps I have taken and am still taking to discover and embrace my natural beauty. More than seven years ago, I decided to wear my hair in its natural state. I share how words and pivotal life events impacted my willingness to claim my own worth.

THEIR STORIES

After telling my story, you can read up-close-and-personal accounts from thirty-two esteemed *Hairlooms* contributors. Each storyteller delivers a compelling, personal account of an aspect of the path to embracing your hair and beauty.

YOUR STORY

After reading my story and the contributor stories, you have an opportunity to write the best story yet: yours. You'll find the "Comb Through" sections of *Hairlooms* directly after the contributor stories. Expect to be prompted to reflect on the chapter material and begin examining your own hairlooms. I purposely set the stage for you to identify and self-correct unhealthy thought patterns. You will be challenged to address open-ended questions about the book's content; this will be a great way for you to explore the next leg of your self-acceptance journey.

Action steps always help me make sense of what I just read. Once you read the chapters, stories, and "Comb Through" sections, the "Strand Strategy" is next. After looking at my own life, reviewing my blog comments, and personally surveying more than 200 Black women, I created this set of how-to steps from some of the most popular topics about our hair and beauty. In this section, you'll find practical tips that include ways to be fit and still have a 'fro; how to handle heat-damaged hair; and how to ace a pop-up interview that is scheduled before your next hair appointment!

Hairlooms is rounded off with a great resource index that cites products and services—only those I personally use—that align with our mission of creating healthy self-esteem. Last, and certainly not least: who among us could use some financial wisdom? The "'Fros and Finance" resource is just the place for tips to learn how to be beautiful without breaking the bank.

Well, ladies, are you ready?

I officially invite you to curl up, kick off your shoes, and get ready for some internal dialogue about the most talked-about subject in our circles. Expect to split hairs on a topic that has been divisive. As you pore over these pages, let your hair down—even if it doesn't make it beyond the nape of your neck. Get ready to journey to a place where you can untangle the treasure on your head that creates tension in your heart. This is the place where your hair looms.

What will you comb through today?

Chapter 1

BABY HAIRS

I t was a gray day. Stacks of dense clouds, heavy with a cold, pelting rain, blocked the sun's rays before they could make it to the ground. As Kyle and I clumsily made our way back home from the hospital, our car was filled with an eerie emptiness. Occasional sighs of disbelief and weak attempts to silence tears punctuated the awkward silence. I carried the horror and shame of a failed adoption. I was still childless, and in that moment, the hope of adding a curly-headed baby girl to our family had been destroyed.

In retrospect, I should have known something was wrong earlier on that dismal morning. In the pit of my stomach, I felt as if all of the commotion surrounding the imminent adoption had reached a dead halt. I was unable to put words to my inner gnawing. Kyle and I cautiously made our way to the maternity ward. Once inside, I was instantly energized and hopeful; this wing of the hospital was ablaze

9

with all of the excitement new life can bring. Images of family members gushing over nimble little toes and fingers; visions of pink and blue balloon bouquets; and the sight of parents cradling their armfuls of joy placed my head in a whirlwind of anticipation. I thought, *Finally. We get to see the mother and take our baby home.*

At long last, Kyle and I located our soon-to-be daughter and the birth mother. The room displayed hints of her arrival. Little bottles and tiny diapers were in plain view. We began talking with the mother about how we would officially make the baby our daughter. In the middle of our conversation, I checked my watch. "I've got to be in a conference call for a few minutes! It won't take me long; I'll be back soon." Excitedly, I recall leaving our meeting for the quick conference call.

Within the span of a few minutes, my conference call was not the only thing that ended. I hurried back to the room where Kyle, the mother, and baby waited for my return. This time, though, the room seemed unusually still. I quickly explained it away. I saw the mother quietly study the face of her curly-headed angel. I thought, *She should be getting ready to say her final good-byes. I know it must be tough for the mother, but she promised.* Suddenly, Kyle's words pierced the silence as he asked, "Are you going to tell her?"

Oblivious to any new developments that could have possibly occurred during my momentary absence, I innocently asked, "Tell me what?"

The mother's lips barely parted. Without eye contact, she glibly said, "I decided to keep my baby."

In an instant, I felt as if someone had yanked my dream from my hands and stomped it on the ground. The tear in my soul caused its contents to silently tumble to the floor. There was no need to scramble for my emotions. There was no need to question the answer. There was no need to do anything but quickly turn and leave.

The mother's words pierced like a knife. I had never felt so empty yet full of pain. It oozed from my pores and left me numb. As a professional communicator, it is rare for me not to know how to fill the silence with meaning and definition. On an intellectual level, I knew what happened. My soul, however, couldn't move beyond a state of shock.

As Kyle and I left the hospital and eventually pulled into our driveway, I could no longer control the heated flush of tears. Unable to make it into the privacy of our home, the driveway became my point of release. The tears charged down my face and wearily collected beneath my chin with rounds of dry heaves. After what seemed to be eternity, my mind summoned my body to move from the driveway. My legs, however, stubbornly refused. I sat spellbound. Unable to leave the car, I was torn between what this drive home was supposed to be and what it really meant. Always a creative type, I imagined a sky-blue day with streaks of brilliant orange illuminating our daughter's tiny frame. Each yield sign would have been an opportunity to snatch glances at our satin-haired little princess. Every stop sign would have given me an excuse to watch her tiny fingers escape the warm swaddle of the blanket. The perfectly positioned sun should have lit our way until our family reached home. Try as I might, the canvas of my fantasy remained void of any color but gray.

Eventually, I lumbered toward the door of our home. Once there, the soft carpet on the landing of the top floor provided no cushion for the fall of my sinking heart. I cast tear-filled eyes on the space in our bedroom that had been reserved for her. I was fully prepared to gently place her in the crib at the foot of our bed. No, I had never been a mother. But *I was prepared to adopt a baby girl.* We had already given her the perfect name. I was expecting night cries, diaper changes, and unfamiliar gurgles. The shock of seeing nothing at the foot of our bed but an empty space almost knocked me to my knees. I knew I could master carrying her in one arm as I gathered baby wipes and diapers with the other. I could do anything that was necessary for our baby, but I could not make the birth mother change her mind. I couldn't magically make her keep her promise. I couldn't make her say "good-bye" to her baby girl when she had just said "hello."

As I stepped past this mental tug of war, I thought, *I've got to take a shower. How long has it been?* Evening was fast approaching as the running water covered my body and exposed my aching soul. I unashamedly let my tears mingle in the flow of the shower.

Today, I understand that there is a depth of pain that can cause a rationale to come unglued at its hinges. The crush of some blows leads us to make sense of sorrow in ways that the world deems counterintuitive. For the grieving, these feeble acts are their best attempts at regaining normalcy.

I can admit it now. I secretly hoped that I could remove the stain of the day's events. To my dismay, sudsy lather and repeated scrubs with my washcloth only left my skin raw. When the last drop of water swirled down the drain into oblivion, *the baby's scent was still with me.*

I am grateful that God used time to cleanse what soap and water could not. Kyle rearranged the furniture, and I rearranged my thoughts. Over time, I chose to make peace with the birth mother's decision. With God's help, I steadied myself for another comeback without a baby. The dash of dreams against the wall of reality is never a sprint. Dark days eventually lighten. Burdens gradually lift. My walks through the children's clothing department don't always leave me imprisoned by my past. When children toddle up to me unannounced, on most days my lip does not quiver, and my mouth is quick to share a toothy grin.

I have found that retracing my steps leading up to the failed adoption has been a wonderful way to move on with life as it is. A trek over old emotional and mental territory often unearths the tools needed for full recovery. In the days and months since those painful moments, I have been amazed by measures that I took initially to fulfill my desire to be a mom.

I'm not the only woman who will try to move galaxies when reaching a goal of any size. We all know, or have been, the woman who hides that must-have dress in the men's section so it remains undetected by other shoppers. I, like others, have concocted dim-witted, sneak-a-peek plans in hopes of a millisecond glimpse of a red-hot celebrity crush.

Now, my plans were turbo-charged when it came to my desire to get pregnant and have a child. Marriage in my early forties let me know that I would have to hit the ground running. A former substitute teacher, I readily practiced my momma-bear instincts by championing the cause of unpopular preschoolers who were not selected as jump-rope partners or circle-time buddies. I also remember groggily checking my body temperature in the still-dark morning hours for signs of ovulation. I can't forget how meticulously I took cycles of fertility meds. The designer "steal" from the local thrift store's maternity section was all the rage. If I was going to be a forty-something mom, I figured I might as well be stylish! The navy-blue sheath dress sported faux fur cuffs. Yes, I have even walked through the house with a pillow under my shirt. How else could I know what to expect when I would be seven months pregnant?

My innate instinct to prepare for our baby took on a life of its own. At forty-two years old, I made the most life-altering decision to date. I decided to wear my hair in its natural state. I wasn't certain that chemically treated hair was unhealthy. I regularly endured scalp burns; this repeated, singular incident made me aware of the perils associated with chemically straightening my hair. In turn, I didn't think that a baby could thrive in vitro with this chemical residue in my pores and bloodstream.

As always, the naysayers and "serial permers" met my decision with unbridled resistance. I frequently heard the full chorus of the "I Got a Perm and Nothing Happened to My Kids" anthem. Nonetheless, I was determined that Baby Roseman was going to have the safest possible "womb ride." I viewed my hair decision as my gift to our unborn child.

Now, it's no secret that some gifts are scrutinized more than others. The reaction to receiving itchy wool socks, versus pulling a hot designer purse from the gift bag, would be totally different—the former likely with half-hearted thanks, and the latter with squeals of delight. Some equated my kinks and curls with those practical but definitely unappealing socks rather than the sleek Louis Vuitton bag.

Many times, I heard a friend say, "You need to do something with your hair." Other times, no words were used to describe the curious disgust with my personal hair choice. On some unfortunate occasions, I've had women I know walk over, look at my hair, and touch it with a sympathy-filled, *"Hmmph!"*

Who knew that natural hair was just another proverbial bullet for me to dodge? Emerging from semi-private attempts to conceive a child is challenging enough. As my forties rolled along, so did the questions and comments about an addition to the Roseman family.

It was not uncommon for me to hear: "What are you waiting for?" "You're not trying hard enough!" and "Don't worry. You have time." These and other insensitive words hit me with like rapid-fire questions during a guilty-before-tried hearing. My all-time favorite? "Don't worry, Michele. Sarah had a baby when she was ninety!" Now I'm all for biblical truths, but who said I wanted to have a baby at ninety years old just because the wife of the Bible hero Abraham did? As I reached and passed my mid-forties, I realized that people will often try to fix what seemed to be broken in their eyes. Most attempts are well-meaning but still carry the same sting as intentional digs.

It's been clear to me that being a happily married woman over fifty years old and without children has proven to be grounds for stigmatization. Believe it or not, though, sporting natural hair has been even less popular than that. When I take time to consider people's reactions to my kinky hair, I'm really not that surprised. I instinctively believed that I might encounter barbs and eye rolls if I chose to wear the hair I received at birth—my baby hairs. It's funny, because many internal messages slip past the conscious level. Unnoticed at first glance, these messages and perceptions often color our movement in very noticeable ways.

During my stint as a writing instructor in Bangkok, Thailand, I experienced firsthand how ideas can sneak into our minds without us knowing that they've entered. Toward the end of my trip, I was determined to try food that was beyond my comfort zone. Once at the breakfast buffet, I eyeballed a tray of jet-black slices of bread. Now, coming from the United States, I could only equate this bread with burnt toast. You can only imagine my shock when I discovered that this breakfast offering was black squid ink bread! I've never been a fan of squid, and the thought of eating the remnants of the creature's protective mechanism was more than I could handle. It made me even more reluctant to expand my culinary palate. After several moments, though, I finally consumed the bread, and I must admit that it didn't taste like I thought it would.

All of my deliberation—over a slice of bread—took place because of mental downloads. Past experiences told me that black-colored toast meant a few things. Number one: I had burned the bread because I didn't properly set the toaster, or the toaster overheated. Number two: The bread was now nasty and not worth eating. Number three: This bread should be thrown away immediately. Withdrawals from my memory bank gave me cause to pause. I had never seen black squid ink bread before, but I received messages that danger was on the horizon. This security alert likely registered because of my personal experience and the name of the bread. Though I was not familiar with what was presented, I was prepared to respond in a most familiar way: avoidance and criticism.

Much like this culinary exploration, as Black women we also have the tendency to run from or turn away from our baby hairs. The Benchmarking Company[1] conducted a spring 2016 survey that explored Black women's interests and purchase patterns relative to particular hair care products. The findings revealed that the 188 Black women who were surveyed had an interest in products that would affect their hair in very specific ways. The survey polled this aggregate of women about hair care products that would do the following: provide ultraviolet radiation (UV) protection for the scalp, protect hair from sun damage, and reduce frizz. Of these categories, almost 90 percent of the Black women surveyed expressed that they were "very interested" and "interested" in hair care products that reduce frizz. Products that provide UV and sun damage protection were not nearly as appealing to them. Moreover, almost 60 percent of these women purchase their products of interest monthly, twice a month, or weekly.

Ladies, let's look a little deeper at what the survey findings *really* say about the feelings we may have about our hair. Based on the data, it's safe to say that many of us may be willing to sacrifice the health of our hair for the "look" we are trying to achieve. Overexposure to the sun's UV rays can definitely compromise the health of our hair. Too much will likely leave our hair damaged. Now, the damage may not be readily and quickly visible, but over time, our tresses will show the effects.

On the other hand, it doesn't take a rocket scientist to detect frizz. Those flyaway hairs that won't stay put are an irritant because they can photobomb a picture-perfect hair day. While it's important that our hair is "on fleek," at some point, you may want to ask yourself, *What am I willing to do to achieve this smooth look?* Why aren't more of us concerned about damage to our hair? Could it be that we are running from or avoiding that which can never be permanently changed at the root?

The survey and our personal lives have already answered these questions. *Essence* reports that Black women spend approximately $7.5 billion annually on beauty products. This figure outpaces their non-Black counterparts by an estimated 80 percent. Numerous credit card swipes and cash purchases reveal that we will pay what is necessary for the right look.[2] The unfortunate side of this response is that our desire may throw our finances down a bottomless pit. As we chase this "smooth" phantom, no product will provide frizzless hair forever. At some point—when we get to the last drop of the pomade, glosser, or serum—we have to face the music. We, in essence, are paying to have our hair respond in a way that goes against its genetic design.

Generally speaking, most Black women have curly, tightly coiled hair. This type of curl pattern is naturally more prone to take in moisture and water. The result: our hair will be more inclined to frizz.

These findings played out in real life. I had no history with the black squid ink bread I saw in Thailand, and I also had no real history of experiencing my natural hair for extended periods of time when I was a girl; I felt like the natural texture was something to be avoided. Hair shampoo and style days for me were filled with the smell of fire-hot, cast-iron combs that met my freshly washed hair with a customary sizzle and pop. This process left my hair straight. Later in life, my hair was slathered with products that promised high gloss and frizz resistance in the rain. My only recollection of seeing my hair in its naturally curly state was while "getting it done." My time with my *baby hair* was short and brief. Like an airport layover, I was in that state just long enough to reach my final destination. What was that destination? It was the place where my hair dared to express itself. That was the place where kinks and coils were banned. At its best, the edges around my temples and the nape of my neck obeyed the demands of the chemical taskmasters and remained in submission for the next four to six weeks. This had become my reality; it had become a place where I had no real knowledge of what my natural hair looked like and how it responded. I am amazed at my reluctance to wear what had been given to me at birth. Each attempt to do so provoked the sense that I was treading on a taboo. It has taken time to delete these old files and add some data that is based on truth rather than conjecture.

Hindsight being what it is, I now know why my decision to finally "go natural" was twenty-five years in the making. My brave, elder, and only sister, Sheila, challenged me to do it as a teenager. A quarter of a century later, I was still teetering on the fence of this brand-new idea. Even at that age, my determination to have my hair straight felt like a life-or-death matter. I remember telling Sheila that if I died before she did, she had better lay my edges down in the casket! Like a neighborhood game of Double Dutch jump rope, I knew I had "next" but was afraid to jump in when I had a chance. Little did I know, I was jumping into more than a life without every-four-to six-week chemical treatments. I sometimes felt like I had jumped into a hornet's nest.

Stinging comments about my hair have made it hard for me to confidently sport my natural hair choice at times. Self-acceptance comes in phases and stages. When I was newly natural, I recall preparing to meet some friends. I made several trips to the mirror and constantly checked my hairstyle. Multiple pats to tame my stray ends and finger-twisting my tresses had become a daily ritual. I was still getting comfortable with my new look, and my feelings were super fragile. After mustering enough courage to leave the house, I was on the way to my gathering. I sheepishly walked in the room, only to be asked the following question: "When are you getting your hair done?"

That one response made me want to hide in a corner. My knee-jerk reaction was simple and familiar. I laughed about the comment and continued mingling with the group as if nothing had ever happened. Inside, though, I was ashamed and felt ugly. I wanted the floor to swallow me up. Since that wasn't an option, I smiled and sucked it up like a trouper. My response to her comment pointed to the familiar, complex tug-of-war over accepting my hair. Part of me was irritated by the rude comment. Another part of me completely understood the thought. I wanted to wear my natural curls but secretly didn't accept them. I longed to be publicly praised for my coils but silently criticized my kinks and waves. In the earlier stages of wearing my natural hair, my personal battle often got the best of me. Weakened emotional and mental resolve often showed up in my default haircare mode. When all else failed, I resorted to straightening my hair.

What made me so adamant about having straight hair? Why was I opposed to opening the door to a new beauty expression? Why did it take me so long to address whether I truly accepted the hair that I had been given at birth? Sometimes, the speed of self-acceptance is analogous to the slow drip of coffee in a percolator. You know the liquid will leave the spout. However, the time it takes for full release feels like an eternity.

The glacial pace at which I've moved to accept my hair and beauty makes perfect sense. I've witnessed the effects of searing comments about Afro-textured hair—whether chemically treated or in its natural state. These words do more than cut through silence. They puncture the soul. The world saw this tension play out during the 2012 London Olympics. I can only imagine what gold medalist Gabrielle "Gabby" Douglas must have felt when her hair became the topic of heated debate and discussion.

People worldwide sat in awe as they watched then sixteen-year-old Gabby become the first African-American to win the individual all-around event. However, the brilliance of her unparalleled achievements was eclipsed by an unlikely suspect. It appears that her stellar gymnastic feats were upstaged by her hair. ESPN, the *Huffington Post*, and *USA Today* noted the barrage of biting public comments that defined the decorated medalist's hair as being "unkempt."[3] In response to Gabby's hair, the following social media comments—along with numerous social media rants—were posted on Twitter:

Why hasn't anyone tried to fix Gabby Douglas' hair?

gabby douglas gotta do something with this hair! these clips and
this brown gel residue aint it.

Some would ask, "How can the topic of 'unkempt' hair steal the
thunder of an Olympic champion? Why would misplaced hairs be
more important than the perfectly placed feet of a highly decorated
athlete?" After experiencing countless incidents of negative comments about Black women's hair and beauty, I know the answer to
this question. Regardless of the commentators' ethnicity, their words
speak to a larger issue. These biting words simply reveal a general
discomfort with Afro-textured hair. Gabby's true feelings about
these comments really came to light as this best-in-class Olympian
gave an interview during the final post-competition interview of
her career.

She found herself responding to fierce 2016 criticism for not placing her hand over her heart during the national anthem. Her feelings
about four-year-old hair comments still made it to an ESPN interview, which marked the sunset of her Olympic career:

> I tried to stay off the Internet because there's just so much negativity
> . . . Either it was about my hair or my hand not over my heart [on the
> medal podium] . . . It was hurtful. It was hurtful. It was. It's been kind
> of a lot to deal with.

Oftentimes, the answers to life's most probing questions are not
revealed until the end of an event. Gabby's true feelings about nav-
igating hair comments came to the forefront during a final media
interview. In other instances, artists once labeled "average" emerge
as brilliant, or ahead of their time, when their musical scores and
paintings are experienced posthumously. The hindsight to accurately

discern answers to life's most complex issues is usually revealed after an event has reached its end.

For me, the end of my adoption dream brought me full circle with my true feelings about my hair and beauty. After all, I went natural because I wanted to be positioned for the healthiest pregnancy possible. I was also tired of expensive salon trips to straighten my hair, but I was keenly aware of how chemicals would impact an unborn child. When medical interventions to conceive didn't work, we attempted the adoption route. I continued wearing my hair in its natural state—without much thought—until the adoption dream ended. Had we been able to have that curly-headed cutie as our own daughter, I would have undoubtedly been lost in the splendor of being a forty-something mommy. Placing pretty headbands and sparkly bows on her curly hair would have taken precedence over my own hair choices. Figuring out whether she looked better with a side part or plaits would have surely upstaged any real scrutiny of my own tresses. At this season in my life, I accept that for now, I don't have Baby Roseman's hairs to comb. I do, however, have some baby hairs to hold. These don't belong to the little girl who I dreamed would come to live with me and Kyle. From tip to root, these baby hairs belong to me.

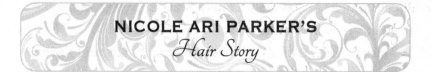

NICOLE ARI PARKER'S
Hair Story

NICOLE ARI PARKER *is a Hollywood actress and creator of the Gym-Wrap, which promotes exercise and healthy lifestyle habits while helping people maintain their hairstyles during fitness activities. She co-starred in the 2014 TNT television drama series,* Murder in the First.

The fact that we were systematically dismantled in our confidence, as a people, is part of the legacy of slavery in this country. I think we have put ourselves back together regarding how we feel about ourselves internally and externally. We are still in the healing phase, and it's important for African-American women to know, believe, and say, "The way I am is enough. The way I am is beautiful." We need to know that the way we are is how God intended.

I think we are slowly piecing together that confidence and certainty that we are worthy and beautiful. I think it's moving to our hair. As a woman with children, I have had to consciously watch my vocabulary when I sit down to do my daughter's hair. I have had to reteach myself. I couldn't say, "Come here; your hair's a mess. Let me do this." I couldn't say, "Don't jump in the pool." I want her to love her hair and all of its versatility, so I had to work on it.

I don't want my grandchildren or great-grandchildren to still be in a sense of fighting and pushing. I want them to have the luxury of choices when picking their dreams, occupations, styles of dress, *and* styles of hair. I want them to have that freedom. Right now I have to teach my daughter to sustain that self-love, so it becomes natural to her. I don't want to force any woman to become natural, but I want to teach my daughter that this is an option. I want her to start loving herself the way she is. If she chooses to blow out her hair so that it's straight (when she's a teenager or I've blown it out for her), I still want her to like her hair in its natural state. I don't want her to view her natural hair as something she has to run from. We, as Black women, have to stop running from ourselves.

It's also very important for African-American women to include exercise in our beauty regimen. I think it's important that we start incorporating a daily dose; we shouldn't try to achieve some ridiculous ideal but just be our best selves. If we could, as a community, wrap our heads around the fact that taking a walk is the same as taking a bath—it needs to be part of your day—then it would improve our health. There would be no pressure to look like a certain person or certain body type. We could be our best, healthiest selves.

On a historic level, we have been through so much as a people. So many generations have sacrificed for us to enjoy the freedoms that we have today; I wouldn't want the history books to say we lost a race of people to high blood pressure. We can't go out like that. We have to rise to our best selves and leave legacies for the generation of African-Americans who are coming after us. I think the last frontier we have as a people is our health. We've fought for our civil rights, and we've really created a movement with our voices. We have to also put our energy behind our health. We're on a journey, and it's not over. As a people, we can't stop working on these issues, because they are keys to our legacy. They are keys to our future. Eventually, though, I want us to be able to "chill" as a people and live our lives. That's the vision in my heart.

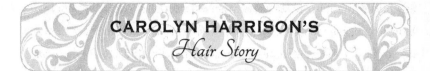

CAROLYN HARRISON'S
Hair Story

CAROLYN HARRISON *is the Metro Director for Young Life in the Greater Bronx. Young Life is a seventy-five-year-old, faith-based organization committed to introducing teens to Jesus Christ and helping them to grow in their faith. Carolyn completed her undergraduate and graduate studies in theater arts at Bucknell University and Antioch University's McGregor School, respectively. She completed a Master of Divinity at Nyack College's Alliance Theological Seminary in 2015. Newly married, Carolyn is grateful for her husband's partnership and creative inspiration. She is most proud of her role as a parent to two young adults and one teen—two daughters and a son.*

I didn't grow up with a father. I was often jealous of my sisters who had fathers in the home and mothers who went to the hair salon every two weeks. That was a part of the ritual, and it was a line item in the family budget. I would see some girls walking around with hair that was moving, swaying, and beautiful; I didn't have that. I do, however, recall sitting in my mother's chair. The hair ritual was something that was not uncomplicated. I loved the results, but I hated the process. I remember getting my hair shampooed, and that was painful for me because I didn't like water in my face.

The results, despite the pain, were so beautiful because she was meticulous about straightening the hair and pulling out the kinks. After the ritual was done, I was sent outside to play. On a particular morning, I was jumping rope. Outside of our apartment, the sun was high in the sky, and the day was beautiful. I was alone. I happened to look at the concrete and saw a shadow of myself. It was six feet tall, and the hair was down my back, and the beauty of it mesmerized me. My braids were flapping up and down on my neck. That was a strong moment for me.

During my first marriage, memorable moments about my hair changed. I wed a man who never understood that ritual and really didn't understand how connected my esteem was to my hair. In the year 2000, though, I had a major paradigm shift that helped me view my hair and beauty differently. I went to Africa on a mission trip for two weeks and was struck by how little focus the African women placed on their hair. In the village I visited, there were women who were living in severe poverty. Some of these women had lost their husbands to AIDS or their daughters to prostitution and the sex-for-food industry. They walked six miles a day just to get clean water.

After this experience, my thoughts changed when I came back to the United States. I remember saying, "What right do I have to spend six hours on a Saturday in a hair salon when my sisters in another part of the world have to walk six miles just to make sure their families don't die from drinking dirty water?" At that point, I cut off all of my hair. This cut, for me, was an act of solidarity and liberation again. I finally had the correct perspective. Whether I could afford a hairdo or not, I was in charge.

I tell any girl or woman to remember who gave you your hair. Remember that all God has made is good. So if He has declared it good, who are we to say that it is not good?

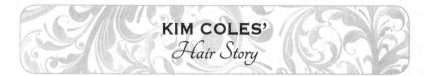

KIM COLES'
Hair Story

KIM COLES *is a Hollywood actress and comedian most known for her role as the free-spirited character Synclaire James-Jones on the Fox series,* Living Single. *Kim has also hosted BET's game show* Pay It Off. *She has also co-hosted on BET's widely popular talk show* My Black Is Beautiful, *which celebrates the unique and dynamic qualities of the African-American woman.*

I come from the world of sitcom. When the "powers that be" build a character, the character's hair is just as much a part of the character as everything else. Synclaire—the character who was featured in Fox's *Living Single*—had a very specific look. When I played Synclaire, if I had started wearing straight hair, it would have looked weird. I had curly, fluffy, bouncy hair that was a part of my character. It was part of the persona; the hair was part of the character.

In the entertainment industry, though, your hair will look different if you're an ingénue or a romantic leading lady. Chances are, your hair will be straight. I think the standard has been set that straight hair is *good hair*; this idea was handed to us by the European beauty ideal. I even hear White sisters talk about ironing their hair on ironing boards to get it straighter. There was a time when freely wearing your natural hair was less accepted, but controlling your hair was more accepted. It was important to straighten your hair and show your length. We have all worked so hard to make our hair look like that. I know I was working hard to get my braids touched up and buy the long hair.

When I was little, I remember putting a towel on my head and then running through the house, trying to get some wind in my hair. I used a little beach bucket, and it was just the right size to sit on my head to keep my towel on. I was always influenced by the commercials during the sixties and seventies. They showcased Prell shampoo and VO5 girls with long, flowing, blond hair. I have envied girls whose hair was softer, longer, wavier than mine. I wanted hair that bounced and would blow in the wind. I've definitely felt that if my hair looked like theirs, my life would be perfect. If I could go swimming without worrying about my hair or if a guy could run his fingers through it, I would attract a better quality of man.

The images of people I saw on TV, movies, and magazines influenced me. I always saw my hair as unruly, unmanageable, and difficult because it didn't do what other actresses' hair did. Natural hair is not consistent; it will look different every single day. Even if you put three different kinds of gel, it's going into be different every day. I think that straighter hair is easier for the hairstylist to control on set and easier to contain. If you're in a movie or sitcom, you have to look the same every day that you are playing that particular scene. At one time, though, the Afro signified a sense of pride. Now, I believe that Black women's decision to wear their natural hair is creating a quiet revolution. We're saying, "I don't want to put chemicals on my hair to look like someone else's symbol of beauty."

When you wear your hair in its natural state, it says to the world that you accept your heritage. I think that for some people, that is a good thing. This decision creates a giant question mark for others. There is a perception that you're Black now. I feel a sense of pride about being able to wear my natural hair. I didn't just go slow when I made this decision. During one trip to the beauty shop, I walked in and had a wig and a hat with me. I left that day wearing neither! I was surprised and happier than I ever thought I would be.

DR. RO'S *Hair Story*

DR. RO *is a nationally recognized nutritionist and regular contributor on the* Dr. Oz Show, *the* Meredith Vieira Show, *and CNN. She is the author of* Dr. Ro's Secrets to Livin' Healthy *(Bantam Books) and* Lose Your Final 15: Dr. Ro's Plan to Eat 15 Servings a Day & Lose 15 Pounds at a Time *(Rodale).*

As a correspondent for a television on-air news program, I discovered that the person who hired me had a different opinion about how a Black woman's hair should look on TV. One time, I got my hair braided before going on vacation. The day after I had it done, I went into her office, and she said to me, "Now what are we going to do about the hair?"

I said, "What do you mean?"

She said, "You're going to be on air tomorrow. It is not permissible to go on with those braids." I still went on the air with my hair in those braids and afterward got my hair done. When I was on the air, I spent a lot of time perming, interlocking, and weaving. I tried all of those options to keep my hair "presentable."

I felt like there was confusion within the station about real beauty. I felt as if the station was buying into a standard of beauty that probably wasn't the best representation for women who looked like me. In general, this standard is based on history. We associate kinky with slavery. Many times in our associations with slavery, though, we have missed the whole point. Instead of looking at the strength of what it took to be a slave, we prefer to see that as a weakness because we have been taught to do so. This focus comes from self-hatred and self-loathing that is associated with slavery. If you take a few strands of Black women's hair, you will find that there are curls and waves. Altogether they may look kinky, but kinky is not negative, even though we associate it with being bad.

My mother passed away when I was nine years old. Her belief was, "You are the best thing since sliced bread, that has ever happened, that has ever been born on the planet Earth. Go with that." I grew up with high self-esteem. Eventually, my mother's best friend became my guardian, and she was a light-skinned woman. My biological mother was a dark-skinned woman. Each were committed to giving me the greatest self-esteem in the world. There was even a member in my guardian's family who—in his own way— wanted to make sure I knew my worth. This uncle once asked me, "Don't you want to be a blond-haired, blue-eyed girl?" He wasn't suggesting that I *should* feel this way, but he was trying to get to the root of how I *did* feel. He wanted to help clean it up if, in fact, my answer to that question was "Yes."

I also remember another teaching moment from my guardian. Her mother looked like a White woman. She had this long, silky hair that she could sit on. I used to have to brush it. This was worst thing in the world because, as a little girl, my arms were short, and they would get so tired. This would take forever. So one day I told my guardian, "Grandma has *good hair*. It's long and she can sit on it. It's soft. It's silky." She sat me down and told me, "Your hair is soft and silky. Your hair is curly." She helped me understand—around the age of ten—that nappy was the same thing as curly. She didn't refer to my hair as nappy; she referred to it as curly.

My guardian was right; my hair is soft. I had never thought of it like that until she said this. She also told me "There is no such thing as *good* hair. The only thing that's good about it is that it's on your head!"

It is important for us to know ourselves and be aware at all times. Celebrate your beauty, inside and out! Develop your mind, because beauty is relative and fleeting. If you are really beautiful from the inside out, it never goes away. So take care of your body; it is the temple that you have for the time that you are here. Celebrate your hair and every part of you, because all of that is a piece of God.

Combing Through: The Process

This section is where you begin to make a turn and start the process of combing through all of the things that mean the most to you. What you'll find are steps, strategies, and methods that I still use to help me completely love who I am, accept how I look, and understand how I feel about myself. This is the time for you to begin to write your own hair story. This is the time for you to develop and begin to rehearse your own positive words about your hair and beauty—your very own *hairlooms*.

The Combing Through section format is super simple! For all seven chapters, we'll take a look at some basic ideas related to each chapter. Next, take some time thinking about and answering some basic chapter questions. Now, take it a step further by using the diagram to address the main issue, what made it happen, and "now what?" or what you will do next. If you're really adventurous, use the blank spaces in the chart that follows the diagram, or even in a separate journal that you will devote to your hair journey, and identify different areas you are ready to address, the effect, and your solution. Take as much or as little time as you need to deal with your personal discoveries.

To make the combing through process easier, I've included a couple of completed questionnaires and sample diagrams to get you started.

EXAMPLE #1:
Combing Through Chapter 1, Baby Hairs

How do you feel about the hair you were born with—your "baby hairs"?

Now I can honestly say that I really like and enjoy my hair.

What do you like most or least about your baby hairs?

Sometimes I still get irritated with the shrinkage. Especially if I'm trying to get a certain look.

If you had it your way, whose hair would you have? If it's someone else's hair, ask yourself why you prefer her hair versus your own.

Sometimes I still wish my hair was longer and naturally straighter. Ugh. I hate saying this, but it's true.

Describe your feelings when someone gives you a compliment or the "side eye" about your looks and hair.

Negative comments can make me feel bad or doubt myself. It depends on "where I am" that day. Compliments always make me smile. If I'm at a weak point, I may still care too much about what somebody thinks of my looks.

Jot down some kind words about your hair.

Curly, soft, pretty, cute

Diagram Your "Mane" Issue

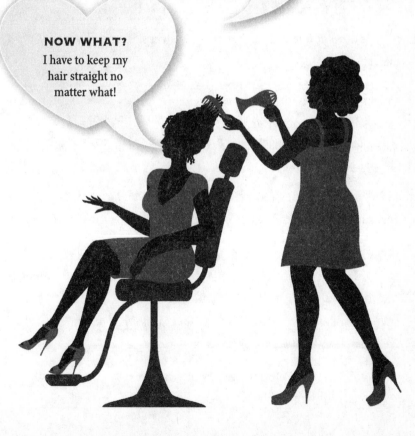

New Growth: Chart Your Solution		
Now What?	**What's the Effect?**	**What's Your Solution?**
I have to keep my hair straight no matter what.	I have heat damage because I use curling irons all the time.	• Accept that this thought isn't true and healthy for me. • Try heatless methods to stretch my hair. • Begin to wear and accept styles that are not straight and show my shrinkage.

EXAMPLE #2:
Combing Through Chapter 1, Baby Hairs

How do you feel about the hair you were born with—your "baby hairs"?

I've always loved the hair that I have. I never had a problem with my looks, either.

What do you like most or least about your baby hairs?

I like the fact that it's unique. I like the fact that no one else has the exact type of hair that I have.

If you had it your way, whose hair would you have? If it's someone else's hair, ask yourself why you prefer her hair versus your own.

This doesn't apply to me.

Describe your feelings when someone gives you a compliment or the "side eye" about your looks and hair.

Either way, I feel good about myself. I'm more concerned about making sure my nieces feel good about their looks and hair.

Jot down some kind words about your hair.

Da bomb!

Diagram Your "Mane" Issue

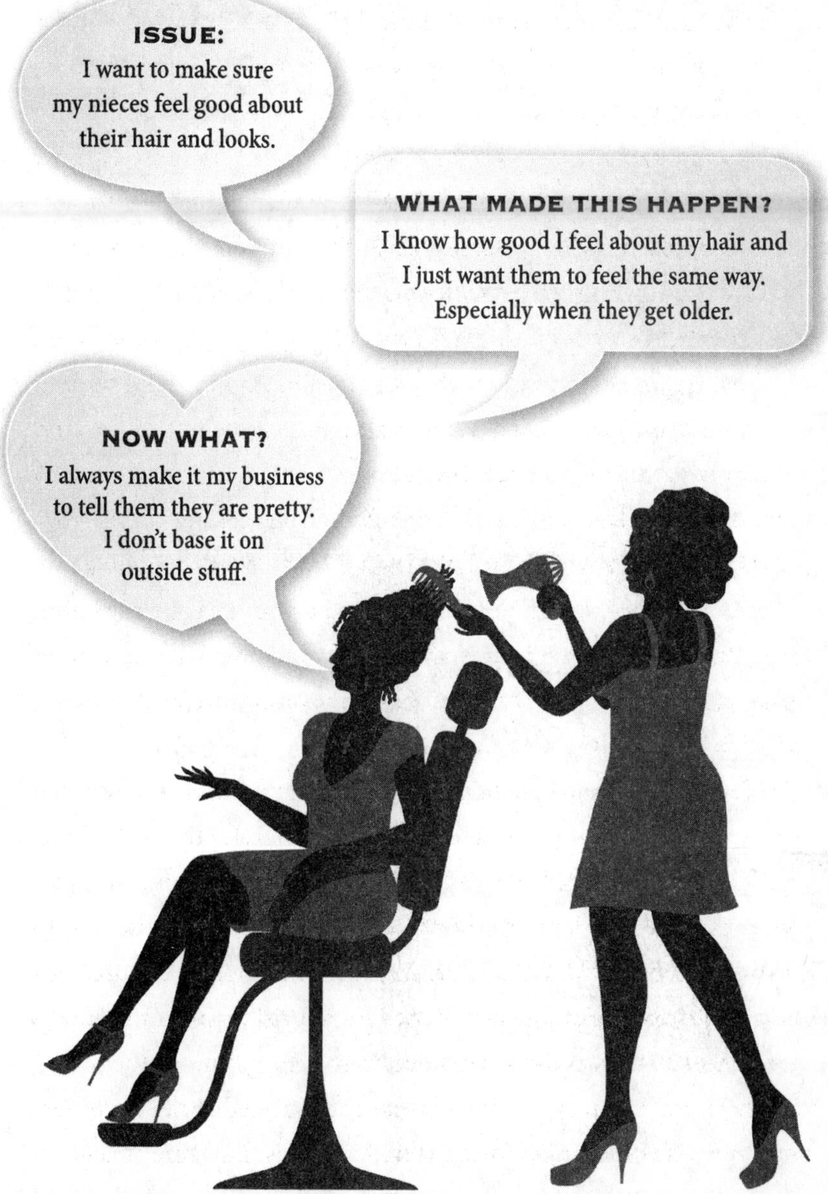

New Growth: Chart Your Solution		
Now What?	**What's the Effect?**	**What's Your Solution?**
I always make it my business to tell them they are pretty. I don't base it on outside stuff.	Over time, I think my nieces will understand that they are beautiful no matter what.	I will keep saying positive words to my nieces.

Combing Through Chapter 1, Baby Hairs

How do you feel about the hair you were born with—your "baby hairs"?

_____

_____

What do you like most or least about your baby hairs?

_____

_____

If you had it your way, whose hair would you have? If it's someone else's hair, ask yourself why you prefer her hair versus your own.

_____

_____

Describe your feelings when someone gives you a compliment or makes an off-color remark about your looks and hair.

_____

_____

Jot down some hairlooms, or kind words about your hair.

_____

Diagram Your "Mane" Issue

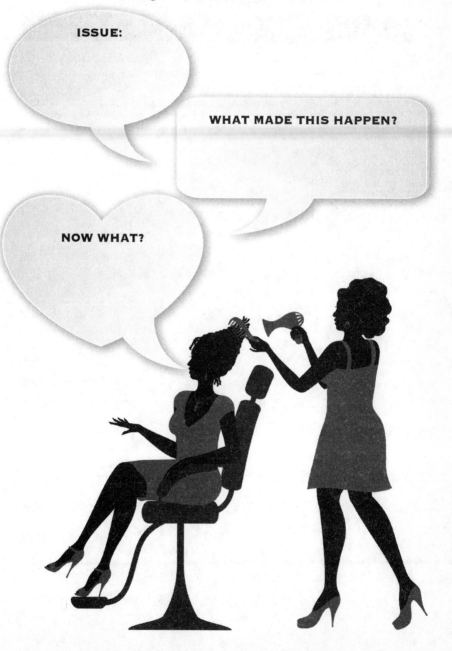

New Growth: Chart Your Solution

Now What?	What's the Effect?	What's Your Solution?

Chapter 2

CHECK YOUR ROOTS

S helly was your typical five-year-old. Her chocolate-brown, chubby fingers spent endless hours trying to get her dolls' synthetic hair to mirror her trademark brown, fuzzy braids. No amount of Jergen's lotion, water, saliva, or Vaseline would create the kink and curl that looked like Shelly's hair. In fits of disappointment, she was known to hastily give her baby dolls the "big chop" and then innocently discover that their hair would never grow back. Shelly's perfectly pink bedroom featured a line of half-bald, knotty-haired dolls. Some even bore permanent marker blemishes on their cheeks; after all, Shelly had to give them the chicken pox when she was sick!

Shelly had a zest for life and laughter. She found school bearable because she lived for the time when she could giggle around the water fountain. Life was all a game to Shelly, the prankster of the family who was always up to something devious. One time, she showed up to a formal family dinner wearing a bear costume. She'd found it in her aunt's attic, so in her mind, it was meant to be worn for the whole family to see.

It was obvious to Shelly, when she was about four or five, that not everyone shared her enthusiasm and zest for life. Pre-K and kindergarten days were great! Other four-year-olds often fought to sit next to Shelly during snack time or meet her for a water fountain chat in the hallway. It was obvious to Shelly that the older girls, for whatever reason, saw her as a nuisance. These tweens and teens had no problem shooing Shelly away with the same irritation shown toward a fly hovering around a mound of potato salad at a picnic. Initially oblivious to the tension, Shelly bravely inserted herself whenever she wanted. Whether popping her head into their conversations or edging her way into their game time, Shelly was determined to be their friend. Her attempts were rarely welcomed and didn't always end up as expected.

A bit clumsy and careless at times, disaster was usually one step away. "Oops, I didn't mean to fall on the puzzle," Shelly said as the teens' hundred-piece, nearly completed jigsaw puzzle was scattered across the floor. "I did it again," Shelly said, resigned. "Oh well . . . I didn't mean anything! Sorry!" Maybe she had knocked over too many vases or blabbed one too many secrets. *Maybe that's why,* she thought, *the big girls don't wanna play with me.*

Then one summer day, Shelly's innocent world changed forever. She was at the park in the Bronx. Kiddie summer rituals were in full swing. Sweaty children ran around wearing ice cream–stained T-shirts; their mouths and cherry-red tongues were dead giveaways that they had licked the last bit of sweet Italian ices. Shelly had already declared in her five-year-old mind that that day, *If big girls don't want to play with me, I don't want to play with them!* As soon as those thoughts left her mind, she was shocked to see the older girls coming toward her. Maybe today would be different. As much as she said she didn't care about the older girls, she nevertheless felt her spirits lift like a helium balloon into the bright, cloudless sky. "Finally," she said. "You want to play with me. *Yippee!*" Two of them slowly moved in Shelly's direction and began to form the familiar playground circle.

Suddenly, Shelley felt strangely uncomfortable. She carried on a hopeful conversation in her head. *They sure are slow. I wish they'd hurry up. Maybe we'll play tag. Yeah . . . that's it. They can chase me. No, maybe I'll be the one to hide this time. We can play hopscotch. Wait, I did remember my jacks . . .* The laundry list of childhood games trailed off, and her feelings of unease grew. The closer the girls walked toward her, the worse she felt. The knot in her little stomach twisted and turned as the circle finally closed around Shelly's tiny body. All she could do was look up from the center of the circle. The bright sun's rays were blocked by their gangly teenage frames. Their shadows now darkened the inner circle where Shelly stood alone. Her discomfort now turned to outright fear.

Within moments, Shelly felt stinging pain in her legs. The teens were showering her with jagged pieces of rock, glass, sticks, and whatever else they could get their hands on. "What are you doing?" she screamed. "Leave me alone! Stop it!"

Shelly's once neatly parted braids began to unravel as beads of sweat formed around her forehead. Her little flower-print, cotton dress was not long enough to cover her thighs and legs, which were now dirty, cut, and bleeding. She was fortunate to be wearing socks and sneakers, which protected her feet. As the barrage continued, the teenagers started to cruelly taunt Shelly: "Dance nappy head, dance. Dance, blackie. Dance, nigger, dance," they sneered as they laughed sadistically. Shelly innocently thought dancing might make them stop, so she made an attempt. Her awkward moves only made the teenagers laugh at her more.

After what seemed like an eternity, the attack stopped, and Shelly ran to the playground's public bathroom. Her legs hurt, and her voice had morphed into muffled whimpers for mercy. The cold, gray concrete walls of the bathroom seemed to trap a clammy coldness inside. Wisps of hair from her two fuzzy braids were pasted to her forehead with sweat. As she sat on the toilet, the heat of her urine stung. While she was relieved to be in the relative safety of the bathroom, she was left feeling afraid, ashamed, and confused. "I can't stay on the toilet forever. I gotta come out. Mother's gonna look for me soon," Shelly said. She wiped herself and washed her hands, "Just like Mother told me to," she said in an awkwardly proud moment. Shelly's feeble push was enough to open the creaky, rusted bathroom door. Her brown eyes cautiously peered outside to see who was around. The rocks were still on the ground, as if to memorialize the day's events. The circle, however, had been broken.

It is safe to say that some things take moments to break but a lifetime to repair. I know this truth all too well. I am Shelly, and the attackers were not strangers, but my family. More than forty years later, I now know that sometimes I have shoved pain into the unconscious places of my mind. Its edges spill over like lingerie in an overstuffed armoire drawer. Unable to close, the contents are always on display for the world to see. On that day, the circle was broken, but all throughout my life, I have found myself drawn to what happened in the park on that summer afternoon. Sometimes, I feel compelled to revisit the gut-wrenching feelings of worthlessness and shame that I experienced. I'm magnetically drawn to that time and place where I stamped myself as "ugly." No matter how far I have travelled for school or for work, a part of me always goes back to the circle. In the midst of job interviews, pristinely answered questions, and well-choreographed moments, I can go back to the circle. What happened there has lingered in my psyche. Vestiges of remorse and shame have never paid airfare but have been stowaways as I've flown across continents. Fleeting moments of success and awkward grasps for beauty are still yanked by the circle's dangling cord.

We as women know what it is like to look up from life and realize that we have forsaken our roles as leading ladies for shell-like understudies. Try as we might, the trepidation to step forward at the curtain call is difficult if there is a chance of being ostracized for things that are uncontrollable. The alternative is often more attractive; some of us, as Black women, only deal with the understudy who has rehearsed the lines but can never live them. The leading lady is inside but struggling to make her debut. My polished, public appearances have often masked the root of sheer feelings of ugliness. No cosmetic can cover a soul's scars. I have clamored for that which is on the surface but struggled to go deeper. I have located beauty in everyone else. When the mirror is turned in my direction, though, I have pinpointed every single flaw I see in myself.

I'm healed enough to know the genesis of my self-scrutiny. I'm aware enough, now, to know my roots. Trees don't thrive on their fruit; they live based on their roots. Roots mingle with slimy earthworms and gritty dirt. Human traffic treads upon these roots. This sinewy underground railroad is all but forgotten, yet reaches deep wells of water that provide much-needed refreshment. Roots are responsible for making God's masterpieces strong enough to tower multigenerationally.

A while ago, my husband Kyle opened the car door for me once we got to church. I wasn't exactly sure why, but he couldn't get the door open all the way. Still, I was determined to squeeze through the narrow opening. I knew I needed to start losing weight, but I was prepared to show the door and Kyle that I could make it out of the car. My husband tried to help me out, but it just wasn't working, so he decided to move the car to a spot that allowed me more "breathing room." After I successfully made it out through the now fully opened door, Kyle remarked that the car door wouldn't open because it was blocked by a tree root protruding from the ground. Now, there were a couple of ways this root could have been handled. If we had more time and wanted to mimic Paul Bunyan, we could have dug up the root and solved the problem. While we were armed with the Sword of the Spirit—a metaphor for the Bible—we didn't think to pack our axe that day! Neither of us had the tools to really deal with the root, so we just moved past it.

At some point after my forty-five-year-old "root issues" surfaced, it became obvious that my definition of my personal beauty began to expand to feelings about my hair. My thought pattern was simple and logical: if I'm not pretty, then nothing about me is pretty. Over the years, though, I have been busy building a career, finding love, and meeting deadlines. I never took time to deal with roots until a time in my life came when I couldn't go through the doors that were opened for me. Moments of low confidence or out-of-bounds arrogance told me that there was a root somewhere. Everyone needs a compliment or has to have a cheerleading squad once in a while. I found myself using people and projects to provide inner refreshment; there was a root somewhere.

Now you and I know that addressing some areas of life is going to take work. Root-pulling requires more than a fingernail file or an emery board. Paraffin treatments and hot stone massages won't fully smooth over the pain of calloused emotions that have toiled beneath a life full of entanglements. Kyle's love didn't help me deal with the root but actually made it easier for me to avoid it. Hindsight being what it is, I asked myself, *How could he help?* I gave him my heart in marriage, but the roots are all mine and could only be pulled by my hands.

As I dare to fast forward to the seconds and minutes of this self-defining moment, I now understand the root causes of my hair responses. I never really understood why I was so obsessed with having long, straight hair. When I started checking my roots, I realized that the event in the park with my family was not a walk in the park. Alternatively, it shaped my view of my own beauty. I emerged believing—without equivocation—that something was inherently wrong with the way I looked. I don't remember reading about the levels of degradation associated with the words "nappy head" or "nigger." My young mind instinctively grasped the fact that they were not the kindest or nicest names to call someone. Their actions told me that my physical appearance was beyond repair. I think I secretly hoped that I would get a break for the name-calling about my looks. No matter how much candy I shared or how many times I offered chances to play with dolls, the names kept coming. It seemed that no part of me was off-limits. I already felt bad about the color of my skin, which was obviously visible. Over time, my ear-to-ear grin was a point of attack. Why? Once my little lips gave way to a signature smile, my hyper-pigmented gums were exposed—yet another fault to be highlighted. Negative comments about my dark complexion followed me into second- and third-grade years. The elation of joining the ranks of the Brownies as a second-grader was immediately eclipsed as they reminded me that I was actually a Girl Scout "Blackie." Sticks and stones did not break my bones, but they did break my spirit.

As a preteen and teenager, I can recall the shock and cautious hopefulness after receiving compliments about the length and straightness of my hair. These comments were kindly and gently shared. Comments like "Your hair is long. Don't ever cut your hair" and "Your long, straight hair is pretty" began to challenge my thoughts about myself. Hungry for acceptance, I quickly surmised that my true beauty was based on my hair being long and straight. My two new truths were simple and time-tested. My first truth: I am pretty because my hair is long. My second truth: if I ever cut my hair, I will be ugly.

These thoughts crystallized as I moved toward womanhood. As if it was yesterday, I recall getting into the elevator of my family's apartment building with a young Black man who also lived in our building. He took one look at me and said, "You sure have long hair for a dark-skinned girl. Watch it all break off!" I ignored the fact that his expectation was for me to eventually be bald as an eagle. In my eyes, he had complimented my hair! Backhanded and all, these and other words about my hair sealed the deal for me. Assuring glances and glowing statements left me with the impression that my hair was the cornerstone of my beauty. For much of my youth and early adulthood, my hair dangled down my back and closely resembled what I saw on television and in the movies. I can recall the pride I felt when I would catch my reflection in the New York City store windows. A glance showed that my ponytails and braids touched the upper part of my back. I was willing to hunch my shoulders so that my hair could creep further down my back. Posing for pictures was a way to strategically showcase my long locks; I would always position my head to allow my hair to hang as far down as humanly possible.

In my dogged determination to maintain my personal beauty standard, I tried every product under the sun to straighten it. If my edges even tried to kink up, against conventional wisdom I would press them down with a smoking-hot curling iron. Even if my hair wasn't clean, it needed to be straight. It was what I had to do. I was a like a junkie in search of the next high. The next high was to achieve straighter and longer hair. I opted for glued-in tracks at the nape of my neck. After all, that's where my hair had become shortest after years of perms. Once I removed the poorly applied track, more of my hair came out along with the track!

I was willing to deal with loss as long as I achieved length and straightness. When I was a young girl, I recall sneaking into my mother's bathroom and attempting to straighten my puffy hair with the hot comb. In my young mind, this should have been an easy task. How many times had I seen Mother straighten my sister's hair or my hair on Saturday afternoon before Sunday church? It looked simple enough. All I needed was hair grease, a steady hand, and the ability to hold down my ears. Little did I know that I also needed to pay close attention to the temperature of the straightening comb. This cast-iron straightening comb was well-acquainted with our hair. The familiar crackling sounds let us know that the comb was ready to undergo another round of the straightening ritual. As acrid smoke filled the kitchen, girly dreams of my debut as magazine cover girl were rudely interrupted as Mother reminded me to sit still so I wouldn't get burned.

After years of this Tapp family tradition, surely I was ready to go it alone. Away from the watchful eye of my sister and mother, I snuck into the family bathroom to straighten my puffs of hair. I had the hair grease. I knew how to hold my own ear. I had the now-faded cloth that was used to snatch excess heat from the straightening comb. All I needed was the actual hot comb. Common sense should have told me that the only reason why the black, metal comb had turned white was that it was entirely too hot. Unmoved, I stealthily closed the door to the family bathroom and boldly faced the mirror. As I placed the white-hot comb against my dark hair, I saw instant results. Immediately, my hair underwent a three-step process before my very eyes. It was straight. It changed colors. It was burned! As I waved goodbye to about three inches of charred strands, I was still grateful because I still had some hair left and it was straighter than straight.

My automatic responses to my hair and desire for length have proven to be a shaky foundation over time. I recall the excitement when I came home from day camp and announced to my mother that I would be featured nationwide in a toothpaste commercial. Reflecting on the casting meeting, I recall being the only Black girl. Over time, I wondered whether I had been selected based on my brilliant smile or my long ponytails. Similar thoughts darted across my mind when I was the only person selected from my post-graduate class as spokesperson for a nationally distributed newspaper commercial. In my early twenties, I was aware that my hair was quite long in comparison to that of other Black, female students. Within myself, I again wondered, *Was I actually considered because my hair had the "look" that was needed? Would I still have been favored had my hair been short and natural?*

Sometimes we women are too afraid to acknowledge that we have moved in waters that are too shallow. We can't admit that what is on our heads has been more important to us than what resides within our hearts. Too often, we have betrayed ourselves for the fleeting pat on the back, whistle from a stranger, or round-the-way acknowledgement. But unchecked roots always have a way of invading character and filling souls with wearisome pain. The roots speak when we refuse to move beyond painful memories that are pressed like withered roses between the pages of our life chapters.

James Weldon Johnson penned the poem-turned-song, "Lift Ev'ry Voice and Sing"[1] in 1900, which was birthed from the parched soul of a people who had firsthand knowledge of what it meant to be emotionally, spiritually, and physically weary. Many Black slaves were sore and tired from the residual effects of systematic enslavement that treated humans like commodities whose bodies and spirits were deemed surplus and who were only valued for what they could produce for the slave owners. In the midst of a system that sought to break the body and bind the spirit, the Negro National Anthem was written. It is emblematic of the struggle that we have endured as African-Americans. I can only gather that these sentiments were perched atop weights that those of us in the twenty-first century have only seen in our minds' eyes. The depth of their deeply rooted pain was heard while many marched in Montgomery, Alabama. As screams of anguish were hurled against the deafening silence of many in our nation, the swell of this song provided a momentary salve as we collectively began to heal. Within the timeless lyrics, there is an excerpt in this song that reveals the soul's escape hatch:

"God of our weary years, God of our silent tears . . ."

When left unchecked, weariness always gives way to tears. Some tears don't run from our eyes but stream from our souls' pores in fits of anger and bouts of rage. No doubt, tears shed in silence have allowed us to endure pressure-filled lives. They have provided expression within the inner sanctum. With this truth as a backdrop, there is a question that hovers around tattered tissues and swollen, bloodshot eyes. What is at the root of many of the sorrows that we and other Black women face? Our smiles are often reduced to tears when our beauty and hair are called into question.

For years, some Black women have responded to this question by traipsing through life in search of "true" beauty. We have clung to and continue to grip images that have been colored by artisans who barely knew our worth and were ill-acquainted with our frames. Notions that our beauty is nonexistent, or forever marred by its mere existence, has left many of us emotionally and psychologically bankrupt. We find ourselves ambling through life with the awkwardness of a teenager in first-time pumps—looking like an adult on the outside but not feeling confident enough inside to walk with the conviction of one. Our unconscious need for public and private acceptance silently pushes us to the pristine walls of academia, where we often graduate with high grades—and low esteem. This pursuit of a sense of worth leaves many of us lurking in the shadows of darkened board rooms. It is here that we may be willing to work eighty-hour weeks in exchange for a pittance and the smallest portion of the esteem we've lost along the way. The thirst for beauty has left the lips of our femininity cracked and parched as we have climbed from familiar beds of addiction and vices. As Black women, we have groped in the darkness for self and beauty. We have checked in every place imaginable and unfathomable. But when will we check our roots?

Roots can reveal history and give us a forecast into the future. Not many of us get our hair prepared for chemical treatments without first checking the roots. One look at this part of the hair reveals its ability to withstand rigorous chemical treatments. This part of our hair reveals whether we've adequately covered the tell-all silver strands. Women can detect the amount of new growth from the root level. Roots determine whether the day will include singing in the rain or swinging past the gym on the way home. Since my journey began, I have started getting to my root issues. My process can be summed up with the following acronym for R.O.O.T.S:

Realize Others Have Hair and Beauty Issues

I was reluctant to deal with hair and beauty because I thought I was alone in my quest. Regardless of where I have been, I've discovered that all women are concerned about hair. Dating back to China's Ming Dynasty, fourteenth-century women were valued for their ornate hairstyles. In Australia, people who are blessed with wonderful red hair are ostracized and colonized. Some Caucasian women with straight hair get perms because they want to have curls, and conversely some women with curly hair get keratin treatments because they want straight hair. Hair issues clearly cross racial and ethnic lines.

This truth became crystal clear during the beginning stages of wearing my natural hair. Countless strangers would approach me for candid "How do you do your hair?" or "Why are you natural?" conversations. I've also had an equal number of conversations with Black women who proudly rock straight hair but struggle with exercise options or complain about their hairdresser being double- or triple-booked for appointments.

As I realized that my secret hair issues were really not a secret, I breathed a sigh of relief. As I took the time to comb through what were some apparent flaws in my own mind, it was easier to be kind to myself. When I flipped through magazines and read how several Black women have conquered the fear of the 'fro, my heart decelerates. My friend's plan to wear bantu knots at a conservative meeting helped me to see a work in progress. I knew that my roots were all my own, but I was not the only one doing some untangling.

One Issue at a Time

Okay. I would have surely lost my mind by now if I focused consistently on every root issue I have with hair and beauty. If I did this 24/7, I'd have an invitation to a padded room very shortly! After I started dealing with the aftermath of the stoning incident from my childhood and earlier reactions to my appearance, my thoughts and emotions were in turmoil. To make matters worse, instead of giving myself comfort and self-love, I blamed the victim; I got mad at myself and beat myself up for not moving on after almost five decades.

Once my fury came down several notches to a simmer, another idea entered my thought process. My alternative way of thinking is best illustrated with a story about how I shampoo my natural hair. While I now love my hair, I hate the process of washing it as it grows longer. Combing through all of my hair and working through the tangles takes a long time. After battling with snarls and knots, by necessity I started dealing with my hair in sections. It became more manageable—and the process far less unpleasant—because I created bite-sized portions.

Bringing closure to many of these feelings has been a work in progress. My journey toward self-acceptance taught me the power of dealing with one emotion at a time. During the course of my healing, once I identified the most dominant emotion, I would then work through it like well-conditioned curly strands. I combed all the way through my issues until I reached the root. It has been said that "The best way to eat an elephant is one bite at a time." I prefer this saying: "The best way to check your root issues is one strand at a time."

Optimize Each Experience

I will never forget my first perm in the nation's capital. Fresh out of grad school, I was seated in a trendy salon. I remember telling the stylist that my hair was not very coarse and that I needed a touch up. She acted as if she heard what I shared and proceeded to process my hair. Within seconds, I felt like my entire scalp had experienced the apocalypse! I can't even begin to describe the searing pain and intense heat that engulfed by scalp as she applied the relaxer to my hair. My forehead broke out in a sweat, and I felt like my life was going to end in her chair. After the relaxer had been washed out, a scab that was the size of a quarter quickly formed on my scalp. How did this happen? She had used a super-strength relaxer on my "non-coarse" hair. Despite the pain and second-degree burn this relaxer gave me, it created the optimal, or highest level of straightening results.

I have made it a personal goal to exceed my expectations when dealing with my root issues. When I had to deal with the root that was blocking the car door, I was willing to squeeze my way through the partial opening. This approach is not optimal but speaks of using minimal effort. If I had taken time to deal with the root, I could have proceeded through a larger opening. That relaxer experience remains etched in my mind. It helped shape my personal pledge to optimize my chances and straighten out the core issues in my life. After all, I don't want any roots blocking my open doors.

Train Your Thoughts

We've all experienced random thoughts that sneak into our heads and hijack our resolve: *Go ahead. Eat the pint of ice cream. You can work it off later. The dress is on sale, so that makes it a smart investment.* From the silly to the serious, our minds are a hotbed of nonstop conscious and unconscious activities. Wedged in between common and uncommon mind play, ideals about our hair and beauty are sure to bubble up to the surface.

So let me ask: What are the last thoughts that you had about your hair? For a split second, what did you *really* think about your new lipstick choice, your fit in those skinny jeans, or the way he looked at you?

It's amazing because, as Black women, we typically believe we can train anyone or anything. Our coworkers know how much personal space we need in our shared office. The men in our lives know what to say and what not to say about how much weight we have or have not gained. The young folks in the family already know how to act when they're with us in public. Our environments are strategically trained—or so we think. If you and I are *really* that disciplined with our external worlds, why are our internal worlds so chaotic? How come we don't challenge our own thoughts about our personal hair and beauty when they "cross the line"? How can we speak to ourselves with such anger and rate our appearances beneath everyone else's when we'd never consider speaking that way to someone else?

The good news is that it is possible to make a thought back up and leave before it takes up residence. For instance, consider this illustration. My neighbor has a new dog—a dark chocolate and black gumdrop-spotted puppy. I have a "respectful fear" of dogs but found my heart warming to this little guy who, like our thoughts, at times rambunctiously wandered all over the yard and through the easy-access fence that separates our houses. As time progressed, my neighbor started training the dog; once he gave a command, the puppy obediently crossed back over the line.

The same principle holds true for us. When our thoughts attempt to go off course—like the puppy—our own words have enough power to bring them back in line. Once we are intentional about switching our thoughts, when we realize we are in command, we can then begin to find a suitable replacement that will help us comb through any issues we are facing.

Set Time to Untangle

I am an early riser and have a reputation for starting my day when the birds do. Clearly, there is an advantage to getting up before the sun does. I have an opportunity to seize the day and finish projects before most of the world arises. There is one downside; when people know you get up at the crack of dawn, they expect you to start working at daybreak. I have learned that to keep my world from resembling chaos, I have to straighten out my day as my feet touch the bedroom floor. A morning for me is never complete without prayer and Bible reading. I will then take some moments to see "how I'm doing." I spend time with Kyle, and then I face the outside world.

I have to make my personal world a priority before I make my public world a promise. I have to take the time to make my root issues first on my list. I know you've got to tweet and meet, but you also have to spend quality time with yourself. Women need to know that hours with spouses and children are essential, but the only way to straighten the outside is to make time for our own inner work. We can get clear when we take time to unwrap what has been packed in our souls. Roots left unattended will wrap themselves around all sorts of things underground. Some issues that we as Black women face have become intertwined with unrelated issues. This entanglement could have been avoided by being intentional about addressing issues.

Remember that our freedom is based on how we treat our root causes. Some of us will take the time to detangle our kinks with a chemical. Others will opt for a gentler solution and tie them down at night. Whatever the preferred method, we Black women owe it to ourselves to be free. There are challenges as we move in this direction. It's not enough for us to just focus on handling root issues. The path we take to our freedom is equally important and will determine how quickly we'll reach our destination.

A literal interpretation of this thought also rings true for me when I think about a particular travel mishap that occurred a few years ago. It is clear that of all the senses I possess, I seem to have been shortchanged when God was handing out the sense of direction. I am woefully inadequate in this area. If I come to a T intersection and have the choice of going one way or the other, I invariably choose the wrong way, much to the amusement of my friends and family. One of my more memorable travel mishaps happened at the most inopportune time. I was scheduled to attend a meeting in Biloxi, Mississippi. I was an essential team player for this particular project, since I had landed press coverage for an event and was expected to produce a live social media feed. I was prepared to hit the ground running and anxiously looked around for the ground transportation that I had scheduled once I landed at the airport. *Strange,* I thought, *the waiting area is so empty. Maybe my colleagues are on different flights.* Fifteen minutes went by, and then thirty, with no new arrivals. I sensed that a problem was brewing, as I was still the only person waiting to be whisked away to the host site. I knew to expect a crowd of emergency responders who were waiting to hear conference remarks from the US Department of Homeland Security Administrator.

However, when I arrived, the airport's ground transportation area was eerily quiet and empty. With time ticking away, I asked an airport attendant about the cost of a cab ride to the hotel. I figured that I would just pay a few extra bucks and get the show on the road. My jaw dropped when he calmly informed that the cab ride to my final destination would be $300. Then it hit me; this was not a case of hyperinflation, but the frightening realization that I had booked a flight to the right state but the wrong city. I was in Jackson, not Biloxi—which was 165 miles away. I had been so focused on reaching my final destination that I didn't pay close enough attention to the particulars of how to get there—like a connecting flight.

What transpired in the next moments was nothing short of a whirlwind. I called my husband and told him that I made a "tiny mistake" in my travel calculations, and now I was miles away from the host site. After renting the first available car and negotiating reimbursements with my manager, I sped to a local discount store. Why? All these phone calls had drained my cell phone battery, and now I needed a car charger. As I scurried toward the checkout counter, I asked a store manager about my anticipated drive to Biloxi. "That's about three hours, ma'am. Just head south as far as you can go," he said calmly. With the same level of nonchalance and a twinkle in his eye, he cautioned me, "Just don't drive too far south, or you'll end up in the Gulf of Mexico." My geographically challenged mind only heard the words "Mexico" and somehow skipped the water part, as I conjured up images of a Mexican guard issuing me an act of clemency for mistakenly crossing the border. I was prepared to use my best Spanish accent and sob story to stave off any accusations of spying.

The sun quickly set as the dark night enveloped my tiny rental car. I prayed, talked to myself to stay awake, and wondered how I could have made such a blunder. Through it all, my little car chugged along without fail. When I finally arrived in Biloxi, I was so grateful that I could have kissed the ground.

Who would have known that putting all of my focus on the destination without considering the route would cause me to totally miss the best path? How we decide to unbraid our tangled hair issues and roots will determine our degree of liberation. The path toward healthy images may be littered with obstacles. As Black women, we may find ourselves paying exorbitant costs with our emotions because we have rushed past root issues. The thought of wearily driving along narrow roads that have been darkened by battered images and harsh words is difficult. Convenience may even call some to pump the brakes on self-discovery. Courage, however, issues a clear call to women who will go along for the ride. This journey may not include reimbursements for expenses incurred. Safe arrival, though, will more than pay for what is lost along the way. Once we honestly deal with the genesis of hair issues, we are prepared to face our fears.

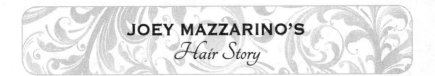

JOEY MAZZARINO'S
Hair Story

JOEY MAZZARINO *is a Muppeteer and lead writer for* Sesame Street. *Joey wrote the "I Love My Hair" song for his adopted Ethiopian daughter. It subsequently became a viral Internet video sensation with more than 6 million YouTube hits. On* Sesame Street, *Joey has performed a number of characters, which include Murray and Stinky the Stinkweed. In 2010, Mazzarino won an Emmy Award for Outstanding Performer in a Children's Series for his performances of Sesame characters Murray, Stinky, and Blogg.*

I have a daughter who is from Ethiopia, and she has beautiful curly hair. When she was around four years old, I noticed her looking closely at my wife's hair. She would put a towel over her hair and pretend to be my wife. After she did this, she was like a glamour queen, and she was loving it. Then she would say to my wife, "I want hair like your hair."

This made me feel terrible, and I would say, "I want hair like *your* hair. Your hair is gorgeous and so beautiful." We had so many African-American Barbies, but she would always go toward the White one and want to do its hair. We were starting to worry about this.

One day, I told my executive producer that I'd love to try and tackle this issue. I wanted to try and get African-American girls to realize something about their hair. I didn't know about the broader issues in the African-American community. I thought it was just my daughter's issue because she had White parents. We should have known the "I Love My Hair" video had tapped into something, because all of the African-American women who worked on the set came down to watch it. Then I started welling up, reading their comments on the Internet and hearing people's stories. The day I finished it, I played it for my daughter, and she loved it.

This experience and other women's responses opened my eyes to a larger issue in the world that I didn't know existed. Because of my daughter's issues—which I thought were personal to us—my eyes were opened beyond this narrow tunnel vision of my kid's and family's needs. I started to think about the needs of everybody's kids and everybody's families.

When my daughter was younger, her preschool teacher was an African-American woman who had beautiful hair. She actually took us to Harlem to find this really beautiful Ethiopian doll that had beautiful natural hair. This played a big part in my daughter beginning to become comfortable with who she is.

It drives me crazy that there is all of this imagery out there that says you have to look like this one ideal. I really don't want my daughter to feel that way. I want her to feel that she is beautiful just the way she is. That's what I hope, and I'm going to keep instilling it in her. I really want little girls to appreciate their beauty and not have to go by what a movie star looks like. My hope is that she will love herself as she is and not want to change anything, because she is already beautiful.

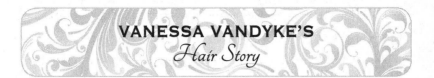

VANESSA VANDYKE'S
Hair Story

VANESSA VANDYKE *is the teenage Black honor student who gained national attention when faced with expulsion from a Florida school because of her natural hair. She is now the "face" of Vanessa's Essence Natural Hair Care, LLC. Vanessa was also invited to share her story as an invited guest on Fox's talk-variety show, The Real. The honor student enjoys playing the violin, designing craft projects, and drawing.*

I feel confident with my hair. I love how it's unique and very big! I also like to draw and play violin, and I have ambitions of becoming a model and an actress. I will continue my education at home and plan to go to a public high school this coming year. My mom just made me the face of Vanessa's Essence Natural Hair Care, and I'm very proud of that. We both want to help young girls like me to love themselves and be who they are naturally. I am also going to be creating a YouTube channel in the near future to encourage teens to be themselves and talk about self-esteem. I will also have fun things to talk about.

I still like to laugh a lot, and I try to keep my sense of humor. An example of this was my time on the daytime talk show *The Real*. I had a blast being a guest on *The Real* along with my mom. The segment was about big hair. My mom and I were invited on the show to talk a little bit about natural hair, bullying, and our hair care line.

If you feel good about yourself, you can try new things and take risks. It's also easier to see the goodness in other people who are different from you or who might treat you badly. You can still hold your head up. You're beautiful no matter what, and you shouldn't change for anyone. I think you should love yourself for who you are. Your choices will decide what you become. God doesn't make mistakes, so why let anyone tell you otherwise?

SABRINA KENT'S
Hair Story

SABRINA KENT *is the founder of Vanessa's Essence Natural Hair Care, LLC. Sabrina founded Vanessa's Essence after her then twelve-year-old daughter Vanessa faced expulsion from a Florida school because she wore her natural hair. Sabrina is also a seasoned marketing specialist who loves to sing, fish, Rollerblade, and make craft projects with her daughter.*

After my daughter Vanessa was bullied about her natural hair at her former school, I wanted to do something positive for her. It was important for me to help Vanessa regain confidence and self-esteem again after this incident. I wanted her to feel good about herself, and I thought the best way to achieve this was to name a company after her. I decided to create the Vanessa's Essence Natural Hair Care line. This company was my way to reinforce the importance of Vanessa loving the hair that she received at birth. While I am committed to continuing this conversation, I am also implementing plans to support anti-bullying and self-esteem/confidence initiatives. My daughter and I continue to participate in the Bring Out the Dolls* charity. This initiative was started because of Vanessa's story.

I also believe that as parents, we must be careful about how we treat ourselves. If we criticize and belittle ourselves, we are setting a precedent for our daughters to do the same thing. So often in our community, I hear parents say things like, "Comb your nappy hair!" or "Straighten your hair to get the naps out!" Even though this may seem harmless on the surface, it can be the beginning of your daughter hating her natural hair texture.

I think that telling them early on that their natural hair is beautiful is so essential. It is also important to help them embrace their natural, Afro-textured hair by using hair care products that will accentuate their natural curl pattern. Let them experiment with different styles they may like to wear that accentuate their textures.

It's also important to teach them about their heritage and the people who have gone before them. Help them to understand that they came from a proud and dignified people. One thing I did with Vanessa when she was a little girl was to point out anyone on television or in a magazine with a natural hair texture. I would point it out to her and tell her how beautiful it was. I think that's very important to help little girls start loving their hair at a very early age.

Editor's Note: Bring Out the Dolls collects dolls in a diverse range of shapes, sizes, and ethnicities and donates them to children's charities.

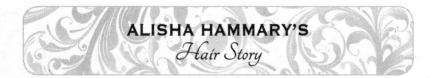

ALISHA HAMMARY *is a senior pharmaceutical sales representative and graduate of Morgan State University. She and her husband Teko cofounded and oversee the New Jersey-based Sportz Farm. This nonprofit organization is dedicated to building character in young men and women through academic and athletic integration.*

My hair is from mixed heritage, but I've never had any issues in my family. I had long hair, and it was considered "good hair." A lot of people viewed it as my crowning glory. If I didn't know any better, I would have thought the best thing I had going for me was my hair. Not my personality. Not my smile. Although I had this "all-fabulous hair," I didn't always feel like I was fabulous.

You know the story of the ugly duckling? That story could have been mine. I had to wear braces on my legs because I was severely pigeon-toed. I had to grow into the size of my nose. I eventually had to get braces on my top and bottom teeth as well. I loved to smile, but I didn't smile so much until I got my braces off, because my smile was just not cute. I had really bad acne, and I was skinny as a rail. With all of these different physical challenges, I didn't have time to think, *Oh, I am the bomb because of my hair!*

At one point, I cut my hair really short. It took a while for me to decide to do this. We spend so much of our resources and time on hair. Some people change their hairstyle every week, and it's completely different. I wonder, "Who are you? Who is the natural you?" I had to move beyond the need to change myself and the notion that I would be less of who I am because I cut my hair. I finally accepted myself and came into my own when I attended Morgan State University, a Historically Black College and University institution. I was able to see all these people who did and did not look like me, but we were all the same. At that time, everything in my life began to change for me physically; this definitely helped me emotionally. Seeing so many Black faces on a Black campus, I learned to be more accepting of what I have. I would think, *All these people are beautiful. I have a big nose, but so what—I'm still pretty!* That's when I came to realize that everybody is beautiful, and so am I.

What we have and what God gave us is great. When you start changing things, it sends the message that *this is not right, so I need it to be better than what it is*. With my little girl, cousins, and nieces, I've always been the one to tell them how beautiful they are, regardless of their hair type. I advocate being the "natural you." Whatever that entails, let it be!

GORDON PRICE'S
Hair Story

GORDON PRICE *is the husband of Carol's Daughter founder Lisa Price and also an accomplished audio technician for* Sesame Street. *Gordon and Lisa have two sons and one daughter.*

When my daughter, Becca, was younger she had definite opinions about how her hair should be done. I could basically do an Afro and work with barrettes. When she got locs, I was able to comb my fingers through them, and it looked like a very neat little mop. Now she has hair like her girlfriends'; she can shake her hair, and it swings. Apparently that's a big deal with girls. For me, it's way easier—just wash and wear! As far as I'm concerned, she looks pretty good!

I want Becca to appreciate the hair that she has. I want her to know that just because her hair is different—it doesn't look like someone else's—her hair is beautiful also. I want her to be happy with what she has and know that it is not, in any way, shape, or form, less than what anyone else has. I want Becca to know she is a wonderful being who has as much right, ability, skill, beauty, and talent as any other creature on God's green Earth.

I admit that I was surprised by the interest women show in having hair that makes them feel good. If they find a product that gets them to style their hair the way they want it, they are devoted. Men don't get it. We don't always understand why you feel the way you do. I remember walking into the house one day while my mother was straightening my sister's hair; I thought somebody had died. I thought, *What's that smell?!* My mother and sisters were sitting there, and once in a while, someone would get an ear burn. I kept thinking, *You all go through some stuff. Why do you care about it this much?*

From an emotional standpoint, I believe that our women have been feeling undervalued for years. Our women generally don't feel as appreciated in media; they're a little more invisible. This can make you feel "less than" and like your beauty is not celebrated when all of the images you see are of people who don't look like you. It makes you feel like, *What is wrong with me? Why is your hair like that, and mine is like this?*

I don't believe this media trend was intentional. I think people just didn't think about it. When you're young, you're impressionable and don't realize these images and words have an effect. You can be harming someone's self-esteem and doing it unintentionally. I'm sure none of the marketing companies wanted to alienate anybody. I think you just don't think about it if you never see people of color. If you live in a place where you only see people of color behind the broom, cleaning someone's house, or performing some other kind of service, then you don't recognize that we're a complete people. We are a whole people with aspirations, dreams, and abilities.

CHERYL BROUSSARD'S
Hair Story

CHERYL BROUSSARD *has been called a powerhouse in the world of business and personal finance by leading magazines across the country. Cheryl wrote, co-produced, and hosted* Ebony *magazine's video* Ebony Money Power, Real Estate Wealth Bootcamp, Ms. Money Millionaire Financial Bootcamp, *and* The Sister CEO Bootcamp. *She is also the former host of the* Mind Your Money *radio talk show, sponsored by Bank of America. A noted author, Cheryl has written several bestsellers, including:* Sister CEO *(Viking Adult);* What's Money Got to do with It: How to Make Love and Money Work in Your Relationship *(Metamedia Publishing); and* The Black Woman's Guide to Financial Independence: Smart Ways to Take Charge of Your Money, Build Wealth, and Achieve Financial Security *(Penguin Books). She has been featured in* USA Today, Entrepreneur, *and other media outlets.*

I didn't feel pretty as a little girl. I know when it happened. I was in third grade, and my teacher did not like me. My hair was pretty long, and I used to wear it with braids that hung down my back. This teacher told my mother that I couldn't have my hair hanging in school because the other little girls would want to play with it. After that incident, I didn't see myself as being very attractive for a long time. I still have issues today, based on that incident. When people see me they say, "Oh my gosh, you're so beautiful." I just look and think, *Really?*

In my home, I never experienced issues with my hair while growing up. My aunt had really long hair, and other members of my family had hair like I did. I felt good about myself because my grandmother trained me to believe that I could do anything. Now, with the outside world, sometimes I didn't feel as if I was okay. They would make me feel like there was something wrong with me. If I had allowed the outside world to affect me, my self-confidence would have been so low that I wouldn't have been able to do a lot of things that I have done. I was able to gain some balance between the outside sound and the inside sound.

I think that African-American women, collectively, have the most profound self-esteem issues in this country. We were raised to believe the messages in society that alluded to the fact that we have to look a certain way in order to be beautiful or accepted. For African-American women, many times we don't see that we look better until someone points that out to us. We really need to deprogram ourselves from all of our old past beliefs and the messages we may have received when growing up. As little girls, we automatically believed that what our parents or teachers said was true. Changing our perceptions is really a matter of affirming who we truly are.

The good news is that we all have choices today. We can wear our hair hanging down, natural, or with weave. We have the options, but we need to make a conscious choice. Don't put yourself into financial jeopardy to have a certain look. Get clear about who you are and what you are in life.

Combing Through Chapter 2,
Check Your Roots

Describe how others have referred to your hair and beauty. Have these words been the same in all of your "circles"?

_____

_____

_____

Have you looked in the mirror and not liked what you saw? What have you done to deal with these feelings?

_____

_____

_____

Have you looked in the mirror and absolutely loved what you saw? What have you done to sustain that feeling or improve your look?

_____

_____

_____

Explore how others' words affect you.

_____

_____

_____

What is a good "next step" on your hair journey?

_____

_____

_____

Imagine you're a little girl again. As an adult, what simple advice would you give "that" little girl?

_____

_____

_____

Jot down some kind words—or *Hairlooms*—about your hair.

_____

_____

_____

Diagram Your "Mane" Issue

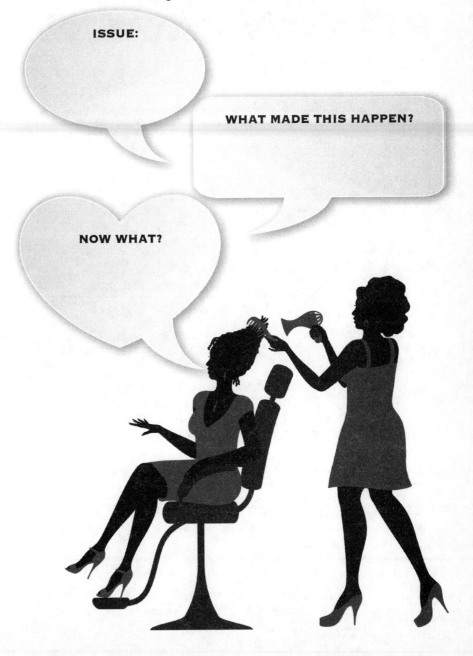

New Growth: Chart Your Solution		
Now What?	What's the Effect?	What's Your Solution?

Chapter 3

DREAD LOCKS

Her handiwork creates knotted stomachs and palms that sweat until chilled. She projects deceptive night images that grip a heart until they're cast in the truth of morning light. With one twist, she has wrinkled many brows and caused feeble minds to race. Her presence drives courage to exit stage left and leaves hope to cower in the shadows. Evasive yet palpable, her thumbprint marks the commoner and the cultured. Recognized by few—but felt by all—her name is fear.[1]

I now realize that unchecked fear, dread, or intimidation may confront us at the worst times in life. If we dare to grab it by the throat, we'll soon find that our ability to conquer it grows beyond belief. The alternative is to live a life that is rendered lifeless in the chokehold of fear. I grappled with this reality during my journey to become a broadcast journalist. I captured my first glimpse of this career vision as an intern in the nation's capital. Armed with the fire and fervor of a would-be reporter, I was primed to excel as a nineteen-year-old broadcast college intern at a local broadcasting company, Outlet Communications. No task was too difficult. No assignment was beneath me. No discomfort could eclipse the shine of my dream job—or so I thought.

I was so captivated by the prospect of chasing breaking news that I lost sight of a fear that was waiting in the wings. As long as I can remember, I have always equated dogs with the three-letter word: R-U-N! All I knew was that man's best friend had sharp teeth and an inclination to leap on everything without warning. Consequently, it was common for me to cross the street or duck behind a car when I saw a canine creature.

Little did I know that the only thing standing between me and an exceptional internship experience was my four-legged nemesis. Words cannot describe the sheer horror that gripped my heart as the producer announced my first internship assignment would be capturing ambient sound at the Ashley Whippet Invitational World Championship—also known as the Frisbee Dog World Tournament.

This event was the place to see dogs furiously leaping into the air and chasing flying discs. While many people would think this was a really fun first assignment, I could not! I only had unpleasant visions of untethered dogs with boundless energy, pouncing on me while I gritted my teeth and pretended to smile. Certainly, I didn't dare reveal my trepidations to the veteran camera crew and producers. As a newbie, you do what you are told, or you risk being seen as trouble from the get-go. After all, there is always a long line of people outside the door waiting for an opportunity to take your spot.

My choices were simple: sink or swim. To this day, I'm not sure how God gave me the strength to perform this feat. The first and last thing I remember was a cameraman yelling at me to follow closely behind as we—on our hands and knees—entered a grassy pen filled with yelping dogs. Canines of all sizes repeatedly jumped over my head as beads of sweat popped out on my forehead. Crouched on all fours, I nervously placed the boom mic near the mouth of a salivating Doberman pinscher. I thought my job was done until I heard the producer gruffly yell, "Move closer!" I took a deep breath and did as I was told. Much to my amazement, I didn't pass out or sustain bites. I completed the assignment and even received a letter of commendation upon completing the internship. On that fateful day, I learned many industry lessons. I also walked away understanding that my decision to overcome my fear of dogs was the key to unlock the door to my journalism career.

Prior to this incident, I would never have been so bold. My uneasiness with dogs made it easy for me to accept substitutes. My first "dog" was the cutest thing I had ever seen. His fluffy, white belly was surrounded by caramel-colored fur. I'll never forget his sharp, shrill bark and stubby feet. He pounced around my South Bronx apartment and was my source of pride. This furry friend came to me with a leash—and a set of size-C batteries. My cute companion was the spitting image of what I'd seen in the FAO Schwarz toy catalogue. Truly this doggie had lots of bark, but definitely no bite!

My decision to substitute a toy for an animal is not that unusual in today's society. Consumers are well-acquainted and quite comfortable with substitutes of all kinds. Those who are allergic to shellfish may eat imitation crabmeat. Some understand that purchasing faux pearls, versus GIA-certified pearls, will keep them elegant and fiscally responsible. Others may inject, fill, or implant if they feel their anatomy is inadequate. Simply put, we accept substitutes when the original is unacceptable or out of reach. Our sway toward the artificial may be driven by social norms or the economy. I truly believe, however, that fear is often the foundation upon which many of these decisions rest. The fear of anaphylaxis makes imitation crabmeat salad a tasty option. The dread of yet another spending mishap makes that faux pearl necklace an easy sell. It is also levels of trepidation that may cause us and other Black women to sidestep the original design of their hair and beauty. Indeed, this fear may cause us to give a nod to the need for imitations.

Now, this rationalization should really come as no surprise. Whether intentional or not, one look at prevailing standards of beauty sends a message that Black women's physical traits are just not acceptable.

If we unwind the hands of time, it becomes apparent that this study speaks to firmly cemented truths that took root well before the twenty-first century. An issue of *The Colored American*[2]—the periodical name shared by two nineteenth-century weeklies—sheds light on this thought. This newspaper advertised the Hartona Remedy Company's Hartona hair product, which boasted of being "Positively Unequalled for Straightening all Kinky, Knotty, Stubborn, Harsh, Curly Hair." The product further promised to make hair "grow long, soft, and straight." The Hartona Face Wash was guaranteed to "gradually turn the skin of a black person five or six shades lighter and . . . the skin of a mulatto person perfectly white." This company's sales pitch ended with a stunning thought for the female reader: "It is your duty to look as beautiful as possible." These references leave little room for doubt about why a Black woman might find it difficult to see her authentic beauty when compared with the artificial standards set by others.

The dread that some Black women feel about their hair and beauty is hardly anachronistic. This age-old discomfort is still a pain point for many. During my six-year trek to comfortably wear my hair in its natural state, I experienced varying levels of fear about my physical appearance.

Fear has a way of dismissing rational thinking. The best and brightest make ill-advised decisions when gripped by intimidation. It wasn't until my mid-forties that I understood how I let fear and emotional instability impact my life. My emotional response to my hair and beauty reminds me of a theme that flows throughout the box office smash hit, *Tangled*. This remake of the classic fairy tale *Rapunzel* puts a modern spin on the story of a golden-tressed princess who is held captive by the sinister Mother Gothel. Mother Gothel fears the power of Rapunzel's hair and decides that the best place for this princess is tucked away in a tower. As the story unfolds, the level of fear that drives Mother Gothel is quite apparent. Though she is introduced as being invincible, closer inspection reveals that this character was haunted by the looming fear of Rapunzel's freedom.

The characters in this story are mythical, but we can relate to their responses to fear. The fear of which I speak, relative to my appearance, was more than a notion. I, too, was terrified at the thought of how I would handle hair and beauty that were allowed free expression. These sentiments impacted many choices that I made about my hair. More often than not, I would see a style that would look great on me. Before I ever was brave enough to wear it, I would imagine receiving negative looks from acquaintances. These thoughts trumped my desire and, as a result, my hairstyle remained the same each year. Visions of wearing twists, braids, and sun-tinted hair colors were locked away in the dungeon of insecurity. I had a poor self-image and tied my personal beauty to the others' comments. Little did I know that my inability to own the rough edges of my emotions was slowly killing me.

I put up a good front for other people, but my soul spoke a different story. At some level, I understood that I subconsciously stifled and covered who I was whenever I elected to view my hair through someone else's lens. Looking back on this now, I realize that my true desire for personal hair expressions was gripped by the fear of "what ifs" that took on lives of their own, spinning off from the original fear and creating even more anxiety and emotional turmoil. *What if they laugh at me?* morphed into *What if I'm really ugly?*, which turned into *What if people don't like me?*, which then became *What if I never get married?* The internal voice of fear continuously screamed at me. Its resounding message proclaimed, "Your worth is tied to your hair!" It implied that setting myself free was really setting myself up for failure; the status quo was working and it was safe, so I should just stay the course. Why didn't I take the leap of faith?

All of us can relate, on some level, to the effects of fear. Some fear has helped us as we've moved from childhood through adulthood—the fear of heights, for instance, protects us from carelessly walking off the edge of a cliff and killing ourselves. Others are irrational, churned up by our minds to shelter us from manufactured threats that really aren't dangerous to us at all. Everyone is scared of something, and the source of fright is different for everyone; while I might not even notice that there is a spider in the office, you might completely avoid going to your desk that day because of it. Certain people, places, and things smother our confidence and cause our minds to go blank. More often than not, this emotion drives us from our dreams at breakneck speed. Unable to escape its reach, we run fast in the other direction—backwards—and crash into the wall of complacency, never living the bold, vibrant lives that are destined to be ours.

Black women, in a lot of instances, dodge hair and beauty fears more than we care to admit. For some, disapproving looks—either perceived or real—and snide remarks have been enough to shut down every ounce of creativity that we might put into our appearances. We ache for the self-acceptance that comes from authenticity but settle for blending in with the dregs of public acceptance. The flame of our desire is reduced to embers and ashes, often leaving us feeling worse because we didn't take a chance. I have often emerged with hair that is publicly appealing but privately shameful.

What Black woman wants to be told her "look" lacks the social or professional polish needed for success? It's hard to swallow the fact that our freedom of expression may impact our livelihoods or our love lives. These trepidations—real or imagined—lurk beneath the surface and often translate into some measure of shame. Shame is the natural outgrowth of self-denial of our personal happiness.

While the measure of our internal worth cannot be gauged externally, a consistently dismissive attitude toward any part of any person makes self-rejection natural. When we deny ourselves the freedom of self-expression, inner tension begins to brew. It is the struggle that drives us to get relaxers every four to six weeks but causes regret when we experience repeated chemical burns or scabs. It is this battle that leaves some Black women with healthy-looking hair but anemic souls. We find that there is a constant level of dissatisfaction with the beauty choices we make. We promise ourselves that we will do it differently tomorrow, but tomorrow never comes.

After deciding to go natural, I opted to wear a flat-ironed style. My look got rave reviews from friends, but I was underwhelmed over time. I got more *oohs*, *aahs*, and social media comments than with any other pictures I posted. That look was obviously a hit. Comments such as "Your hair is beautiful," "Just keep it long," and "Don't cut it" were in abundance. Once again, my long, straight hair was a fan favorite, but I wasn't pleased with my image. The hairdresser did her job, but I didn't do mine. I paid for a new look but paid no attention to my own feelings. I couldn't muster the strength to go after the look I really wanted. The process of developing an inner resolve that overrides fear is difficult and does not happen all at once. No amount of hair pomades or beauty aids will win this civil war. We can only resolve this tension by facing our fears and combing through the areas they have affected.

The process of combing through tangled hair often involves loss and shedding. Knots and curls that don't easily unravel become casualties of the struggle. For the determined, the loss of some hair—or fall-out—is not a deterrent.

The truth is—and all of us know this to some degree—that victory hinges on being able to handle fall-outs that have nothing to do with hair—the disappointments, struggles, and heartaches of everyday life. Our fall-out may have been with a friend who decided that the relationship was not in vogue. Or maybe it is the heartache and headache of a contentious divorce. Perhaps it is the loss of a job that resulted in financial hardship, a pile of mounting bills, and even foreclosure. Most severe, though, are the fall-outs that we have with ourselves. We can find different, truly loyal friends. We can move on after a divorce and find new love. We can find a new job and find our financial footing once again, but we are always with ourselves. Maybe this familiarity is one reason why we are notorious for running roughshod over our inner vows. Familiarity, as they say, breeds contempt. We promise ourselves to wear hairstyles that complement ourselves but quickly renege. We swear to never wear a ponytail to work, but the effort to make our hair look "presentable" in the face of humidity is more than we can bear. We know we need a trim to cut away the damaged split ends, but the desire for shoulder-length tresses makes us push the date with the scissors back just four more weeks.

Relationship reconciliation after a slight or an argument is always difficult. Apologies and promises to "never let this happen again" may placate an offended friend, but how do you make amends when the friend you have hurt is *you?* Since we pretty much never apologize to ourselves, we might binge on chocolate or junk food in an attempt to soothe our hurt souls. That, of course, just makes your body feel awful and leaves excess weight in the wrong places, leaving you feeling even worse about yourself later. Maybe we attempt to placate ourselves with a shopping spree, but trinkets and a pair of new shoes will hardly help us emerge from the mall with feelings of self-worth in our bag. The way to handle a fall-out with the most important person in your life—you—is to pull out all of the stops and make every effort to renew your personal pledge to yourself.

Many times, our personal promises and self-definition are inextricably tied to our desires. Those dreamy longings are often connected with very concrete ideas that tend to capture our waking moments. Every January 1, countless people make New Year's resolutions. You might want to lose weight, for instance, to fit into your clothes again and feel better; you need to make an entrance at the June high school reunion. Your winter workouts during the cold, dreary days will definitely pay off when your winter clothes come off! For me, I was crystal clear about how and why I wanted to express my hair. I arrived at my destination when I mustered the God-given courage to wear what years of hot combs and relaxers had tried to unnaturally subdue. My steps were marked and slow, but each week I made steady progress in my transition from chemically straightened to natural hair. It was, indeed, becoming a reality as I moved away from fear and dread, and toward true self-love and acceptance.

Each time at the salon when I tried different options with my hair in its natural state, I realized that fear was giving way to self-acceptance, and I had fun exploring all the possibilities that these options offered. I began to embrace the fact that my hair is actually three different textures in different areas of my head. At some point, I refused to slather my hair with waxy creams and decided to let it show kinks and curls. I even allowed my hair to remain fuzzy around my temples and at the nape of my neck after perspiring. My bravery turned into steely resolve as I ignored nonsensical questions from peers, such as, "What is your hair doing?" and "When are you going to get your hair done?" In the past I might have said, "I already know. I'm getting ready to fix it in a couple of days," but now, with newfound pride and courage at the ready, I kept my composure and retorted, "My hair is doing its own thing!"

The most accurate benchmark of personal progress and eventual success was my willingness to boldly wear hairstyles that suited me, regardless any past history. I'd always worn my hair bone straight. Flatirons, hot combs, and relaxers dared my edges and "kitchen" to curl in the slightest way. I was the epitome of corporate culture. As I shared earlier, my aspiration to become a television anchor shaped a lot of my ideas about which hairstyles were appropriate. In the seventies and eighties, many Black female anchors blazed a trail for others professionally. In doing so, they wore hairstyles that were straight. I admired and revered these television role models, who also influenced my sense of personal beauty. However, my present-day opinion is quite different. I still have a deep admiration for sleek, shiny looks, but I equally adore styles that are tightly curled and wildly wavy.

My trek from fear to freedom was complete when I made a landmark decision to wear gel twists on the job. I made the hair appointment on the day I was to begin an onsite writing assignment for a federal government grant review. This was a huge step for me because, as a twenty-plus year professional, I already knew the unspoken rule that hairstyles needed to fit nicely into the status quo box. My careful observations revealed that straight hair was in order, but my coily, kinky hair would not be a hit. In hindsight, I think I subconsciously made the appointment close to my check-in time at the host hotel. This time would allow me no "out." I would have no time to change my mind once my style was complete, because my colleagues were awaiting our in-person, kickoff meeting.

The perfectly sculpted gel twists were prettier than I could have imagined. Each strand of my dark brown hair was tightly wound to create twisted clusters that neatly framed my mahogany face. We often hear that your hair is your crowning glory, and I really felt like it was with this style. A tiara encrusted with jasper, citrine, chocolate diamonds, and topaz was no match for my crown of curls. I'd been deliberating about going natural for twenty-eight years, so this hairstyle was an idea whose time had finally come. At age forty-four, the moment just seemed right for my hair to fall freely, with no one dictating how the strands would land.

As I basked in the afterglow of self-affirmation, a storm cloud began to move in from the distant emotional horizon. A knot of fear worked its way into the pit of my stomach, raining waves of doubt on my festive emotional parade.

This singular hairstyle moved the marker for my personal beauty. I had boldly decided to disturb the proverbial stack of dominos. This was not the time for deep levels of introspection and buyer's remorse. After all, the hairstyle was a done deal, bought and paid for. Nonetheless, I ran to the back of the line for another trip on the emotional rollercoaster. Familiar tense moments and tough questions darted through my mind. *What if they hate my look? What if I'm sent home because I don't look the part? Do I look like Buckwheat? What if I'm rejected?* Before I heard from anyone else, I answered the questions alone. I lovingly gazed at myself in the rearview mirror at stop signs and red lights. As often as possible, I told myself that my hair looked beautiful. I assured myself that I would be just fine.

My affirmations came to a halt as I approached the hotel driveway, had my car parked by the valet, and sprinted to the conference room. The pressure was more than I could bear. I found the meeting room and knew that all of my colleagues were waiting for me. With nowhere to go but forward, I shoved open the conference door. My colleagues' gasps filled the room, and their eyes cast fresh glances upon my new hairstyle.

The *oohs* and *aahs* I received at that moment came as a complete shock but a pleasant surprise. I cannot tell you that every professional encounter was the same. What I will say is that my response to my hair and beauty changed that day. Now, whether I'm going to teach a writing class or running to Walmart for a bargain, I endeavor to be my biggest cheerleader. Each kind word spoken by me, about me, boosts my self-esteem and mutes the voice of fear and its emotional cohorts.

What I have penned will take you moments to read, but my journey from fear to complete freedom is taking years. I have made great strides, but there are still days when I have a "game on" kind of day.

My emotional legs are a little wobbly, and doubts attempt to surface relative to my hair choices. On these days, I have to pay close attention to what I call my "wave pattern."

All Black women have wave patterns. I am not referring to how our curl pattern ranks on a numerical hair classification system. There are some things, people, and thought processes toward which we gravitate. We "wave" or welcome thoughts that say we're having a bad day because our hair may not look like we want it to look. Some of us refuse to exercise because we believe outer beauty supersedes the need to maintain a healthy level of blood sugar, cholesterol, and weight. Our responses have become Pavlovian in nature, and we miss the best parts of who we are.

The steps to move us from fear to freedom are easily illustrated by examining one of my favorite hairdos. I have fallen in love with two-strand twists. This style is achieved by using a technique from which its name is derived. Once my hair is divided in sections throughout my head, I take two strands and begin to twist them together. I repeat the same process until my head is completely covered with these creations. There are times, though, when I look in the mirror and I realize that some of the twists were not correctly formed. At that time, I simply take the "two-strand" twist that is misshapen and begin to unravel it one piece at a time.

Likewise, when Black women realize that the strands of our lives have been tightly wound around dread and fear, it's time for us to unravel. A careful tracing of our lives' strands will eventually lead us to the point where the twisting began in the first place. Careful observation of each strand in our life will transport us to a place where hair initially stole the show and became our mane attraction.

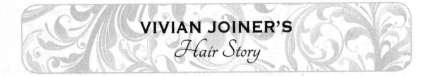

VIVIAN JOINER'S
Hair Story

VIVIAN JOINER *is the co-owner and founder of Sweet Potatoes, an award-winning restaurant in the Downtown Arts District of Winston-Salem, North Carolina. Sweet Potatoes features Southern-inspired food.*

Before wearing locs, I was at a point where I needed to do something different. I needed to do something for me. I worked in corporate America. In the restaurant industry, there was a certain look that restaurant managers—especially if they were Black—were expected to have. Processed hair was very bland looking. I just did not have that look, so I said, "I'm just going to do me." In my early twenties, I went to a hair salon near my job. I walked in and said, "Can you cut my hair?" She cut it a perfect two inches all the way around. I've worn my hair natural ever since.

I eventually transitioned from just a short cut to locs. This has been a growing process. I grew a lot and I found out a lot about myself. I tell people all the time, "If you don't get anything else out of wearing your hair in locs, you will learn patience." You have to be patient with yourself because your hair is going to do whatever it wants to do. No matter how much you want your hair to lay down or your locs to go in this direction or that direction, they're going to do what they want. They will move when they want.

I do remember the summer when I was wearing locs and decided to cut them. I did it while I was away on vacation. That way, I would have a few days to adjust to it and kind of see the new look without having to answer a lot of questions like "Are you sick?" For some reason, that's always the thought when a woman goes from wearing long hair to really short hair. When I cut my locs, I realized that for a long time, people had associated me with my hair. My locs were very long, and my hair was fairly thick. It got to a point where people didn't see me. They saw my locs. People didn't talk about me. They weren't interested in me, but they were interested in my locs, so I was totally the second personality to my own self.

For women in general—and specifically African-American women— you grew up with that statement that *your hair is your crown and glory.* Whether you believe that or not, it in some way influences the way people perceive you or how you perceive yourself. I believe that people may process their hair—a lot of times—to conform. To wear your hair natural is to be focused on the internal instead of the external.

Now understand, though, that you can still hide behind a hairdo even in a natural state. You can hide or change the way you feel that day based on what you do with your hair. When you wear your hair in traditional locs or a short, natural state, there isn't enough to hide behind. People see you. When you put on a colorful top or you wear your hair forward, you can still hide behind the mask of the day. I think that we tend to hide behind ourselves. We are able to put on a different persona based on how we feel that day. Our hair may make us feel short and sassy or long and flowing. Hair attaches itself to the way people perceive you. When we change things that suddenly, sometimes people don't know how to take it. They have taken the persona—versus the person—for so long. At some point as we age, the face that we wear has got to be the face that we are. At some point it all falls away. You can't live behind a mask forever.

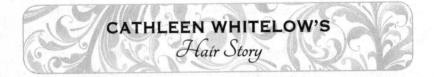

CATHLEEN WHITELOW *is the founding owner of Cathleen Whitelow Jewels. Her works of art have been sold in Saks Fifth Avenue and other high-end retailers. Cathleen is also a skilled corporate communications strategist and earned a bachelor's degree in management/marketing from Loyola University New Orleans.*

In my opinion, beauty in the African-American community meant relaxed hair, long hair. I was already wearing my hair like that when I launched my business, so I wasn't getting ready to change it. At the height of my business—Cathleen Whitelow Jewels—my jewelry retailed in fifteen Saks Fifth Avenue stores, and I was featured on the *Oprah Winfrey Show*. I wanted to have this *look*.

Everybody knew me based on how I looked with my weave, but for thirty-five to forty years, I forced my hair to be something that it naturally wasn't. I felt as though my hair was crying. The more relaxer I put on my hair, I felt like my hair was saying, "Stop doing this to me. I'm growing, and every time I grow, you are burning me off." That feeling was so strong that I started thinking about going natural, but I also wondered if men would still find me attractive and desirable. I was at the grocery store, and one of the managers—who happens to be a White guy— always complimented me on my hair, whether natural or weaved. On one occasion, he said, "Hi. It's good to see you still loving your hair." I had known him for more than a year, and he remembered me with my long hair, even when it was natural. Now, in another instance, I met an older Black guy who had seen a picture of me wearing a long weave. When we finally met after my "big chop," he said that I looked more feminine with my weave than I did with my natural hair! I was shocked because this was an older gentleman. And I thought he was going to say just the opposite.

Over time, I just got tired of going to a beauty salon and spending most of my day in a beauty salon. I just got tired of thinking, *I've gotta have long hair*. I eventually got tired of playing those mental gymnastics, and I just made the choice to change. One Friday night, I went to see a girlfriend who had done my hair in the past. She cut my extensions out. I went home that night, took pictures of my hair, and saw how damaged it had become. The next morning, I went to a young lady who specializes in natural hair care. I went from my hair being all the way down my back to short hair and never looked back. Now my hair is not crying, and I'm caring for it like a newborn baby.

Sometimes what we do to ourselves physically is a manifestation of what we are doing to ourselves internally. Question your motives. As you uncover the reasons, find a way to deal with those issues through church, girlfriends, or guy friends. Once you get peace, you will probably stop doing certain things. To make peace, find out why you put extensions in your hair, relax, or whatever you do to your hair. If you're doing it because you just like the way you look—and you're not tieing it to some deep-rooted issue—more power to you! But if you're doing it because something is going on within you, then deal with that.

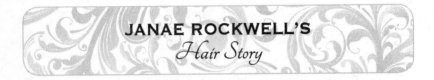

JANAE ROCKWELL'S
Hair Story

JANAE ROCKWELL *is the co-writer of teenage actress-singer Willow's Smith's "Whip My Hair" and a Universal Music Publishing Group singer-songwriter. This single landed a Billboard Hot 100 spot, and its video was nominated for Video of the Year at the BET Awards of 2011.*

"Whip My Hair" was meant to be a dance song and something positive for women in the clubs. It was meant to take the focus off of body image and to unite girls with something we can all relate to.

My hair is naturally curly, and for a long time, I didn't like that. My mother is White, and my father is Black; I had a different hair texture and type than either one of them. I always wore my hair in a ponytail. Then at one point, I had "micros" for the longest time because my mom couldn't figure out what to do with my hair. Even though I was mixed, I was always the Black kid in the schools and in the community.

So growing up, I didn't like my hair. Growing up, I felt my hair was ugly. I felt I was ugly. I was in a community where there were White people with straight, blonde hair. My hair was brown and curly, it was thick, and it was different. I didn't know that it was good. I didn't know it was beautiful. No one in that community ever told me it was beautiful until I stepped out into the world. After coming out of that community, seeing different women with different hair types, and watching how they did their hair, it boosted my self-esteem.

It's been a long, long journey with my hair. I've finally learned how to embrace it. Through the advances in the hair industry, I've learned to use different products and technologies. One day I learned how to wash it, and let it dry and be curly, and embrace it. My hair expresses my moods now, so if I'm feeling free and I want to show people what I've got, I'll wear it wavy. *I love that it's curly and does it by itself!* I'll just put some water and some oil in it and call it a day.

God has given us what we have for a reason. I would suggest learning your hair type. I spent hours in the mirror styling it different ways and playing with different products, but it was a learning process, and it didn't happen overnight. I don't think it happens overnight for anybody. I would suggest studying your hair and learning to love it, because this is what you've got.

DIANE COLE STEVENS'
Hair Story

DIANE COLE STEVENS *is the CEO of Cole Stevens Salon, which is a noted leader in luxury, multiethnic hair care. An internationally recognized hair cutting and design leader, she is also an educator, entrepreneur, and philanthropist. Her expertise also offers effective salon management, marketing best practices, revenue growth, profitability, and work-life balance instruction to salon owners and stylists throughout the United States and abroad. Diane is also founder of the Cinderella Foundation, which is a nonprofit 501(c)(3) international organization, which fosters healthy self-esteem in girls and women in the United States and Sierra Leone.*

My hair was always coarse. This means that the diameter of each strand was very thick. My hair is also very coily. When I was a young girl, I think my parents were more concerned about my hair looking right than even I was. I didn't really compare my hair to other people's hair. When I was young, straighteners were really big, and my family thought that I should straighten my hair. I was fine with my hair, but I did it because that's what everybody did. Later in life, I saw that my hair wasn't growing with chemicals in it. I then started doing my own hair. I never had a problem with the curly hair coming in. I think the best hair in the world is curly hair, because it has a lot more versatility and it looks thicker and fuller. If you have curly hair, you can have straight hair easily. Hair wasn't my concern, and I didn't have that focus. My concern was more about the shirt I was wearing or the socks that went with my shoes. I just accepted and loved what God gave me naturally.

I think the media and parents put a lot of focus on how hair should look, but kids don't know how it should look. Tell them to embrace their own beauty and their own hair. Find a salon or stylist that can address whatever the hair challenge is—not the mother's challenge, but the child's. If the child's hair is frizzy, for example, work at solving the problem. If your child's hairline looks like it's weak or damaged, find a salon or stylist who can address the problem. If the child is a swimmer and wants to solve her hair problem, maybe braids would be a great option. I've also noticed that a lot of times, young girls don't want to get a hair trim because they associate it with getting their hair cut shorter. Parents should implement a healthy routine when the child is young. They should find out what a healthy scalp and healthy hair really means.

I want people to naturally embrace what they're born with and learn how to work with whatever they have. Whatever hair you were born with, make it the best it can be. It doesn't matter if your hair is curly, coily, or kinky. I think we were made and designed perfectly.

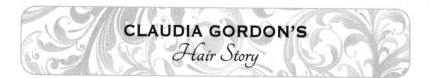

CLAUDIA GORDON'S
Hair Story

CLAUDIA GORDON *is the first Black deaf attorney in the United States. Claudia was part of President Obama's Presidential Delegation that attended the Opening Ceremony of the 2016 Paralympic Summer Games in Brazil. At eight years old, she suddenly lost her ability to hear, but taught herself to communicate in sign language. Claudia eventually enrolled at the American University's Washington College of Law, where also she graduated with honors in 2000 and passed the Maryland Bar on first attempt. The recipient of the prestigious Skadden Fellowship, she has served as Senior Policy Advisor with the U.S. Department of Homeland Security's (DHS) Office for Civil Rights and Civil Liberties (CRCL). While at DHS in 2006, she received the Secretary's Gold Medal Award from then-DHS Secretary Michael Chertoff in recognition of her exemplary work on behalf of people with disabilities in the Gulf Coast both during and after Hurricane Katrina.*

I was born and raised in Jamaica. In Jamaica—I think like many Caribbeans—you find that there is a different standard of beauty for Black, dark-skinned and Black, light-skinned people with curly hair. If you were dark-skinned with nappy hair in Jamaica, you weren't considered beautiful. So as a child I always felt inferior. There was a lot of rejection for kids like me because we didn't resemble what society said true beauty should look like.

When I lost my hearing, my mom married a gentleman who was a Black Indian with wavy hair. At that point, I began living with his family. I was the only nappy-haired, brown-skinned girl in that house. One of the first things they did was cut off my hair. I imagine that they did this because they had no experience with nappy hair. This was very humiliating for a deaf girl at my age. I looked like a boy, and kids had another reason to tease me. It was very clear that I was alienated. When family time would come, everyone would sit down in the living room around the TV, and my cousins' hair would be stroked. I wish someone had told me, "Don't worry. Your hair suits your face." Then I wouldn't have tormented myself.

Now, I think that having my hair natural and cut short is the most professional look I can achieve. I tried everything before I got to the point of going natural. I've worn braids for many, many years. I've permed my hair. However, my hair is not the kind of hair that can carry a perm for more than two weeks. To have my hair looking really sharp required constant visits to the hairdresser, and that was very expensive. It was not just about the money, but it was more about how much time I spent sitting in a hair salon. I would lose an entire day. Eventually, I had to think about now much stress it created when there were so many other things I needed to do with my time.

While I've enjoyed many styles, it was just a temporary thing. When I finally cut off my hair, I felt free. I can go to work in a suit, and I feel very well put together from head to toe. On the weekend or the evening—if I'm going out—I can feel the same way. It's the right hairstyle for every situation, with low maintenance, and it's cost effective.

So I think I've arrived at the place where I've accepted my style. Over the years, I've gotten to the point of knowing that self-acceptance, self-respect, and beauty come from within. So it's really a process.

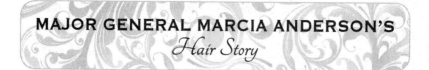

MAJOR GENERAL MARCIA ANDERSON'S
Hair Story

MAJOR GENERAL MARCIA ANDERSON (MG ANDERSON) *is the second African-American woman to achieve the rank of major general in the United States Army Reserve (USAR). MG Anderson is the senior advisor to the Chief, Army Reserve on policies and programs for the USAR. As a Citizen-Soldier, MG Anderson is employed by the United States Courts, where she serves as the Clerk of Bankruptcy Court, Western District of Wisconsin, located in Madison, Wisconsin.*

As an African-American woman, you just have different hair challenges. Sometimes you find yourself struggling to maintain professionalism and not damage your hair. In addition to having my hair braided, at one point I had a Jheri curl, and I found that it wasn't very practical. I've had my hair in short Afros. You name it; I've worn it all. I've been doing this for thirty-five years, and I've had my hair in those styles throughout my career.

About ten years ago, I had some significant hair loss. This resulted from using relaxers.

Over time, my scalp was affected, and my dermatologist recommended that I braid my hair. At the time, I was a lieutenant, and that's very senior in the U.S. Army. I had braided my hair once or twice in my professional career, but I was much more junior and had less of a managerial role.

At that point, I decided to braid my hair because I didn't want to lose it. The results were pretty spectacular. I got a lot of questions about it. Everyone thought it looked great and was very practical for what I needed to do. I was able to educate a lot of male soldiers—who were not African-American— about what it took for me to look the way they always saw me. This was an interesting experience for me, because I never expected to get those kinds of questions or interest. I had established a good professional relationship with them, so they felt comfortable asking me questions. I found that a lot of them had been wondering about these things, and they simply didn't have anyone to ask. They also knew that in some point of their careers, they may manage someone who had similar requirements. These male colleagues realized they needed to be able to have an intelligent conversation with them. My sharing helped them to become better leaders when the time came.

My mother, grandmother, and most of my family members would say that, "Your real beauty is what's inside of your heart and your head. It's not what you look like on the outside." I think too many people think that assimilation means we have to lose a part of ourselves. I believe that your beauty is also the value you add to any organization. Excel at what you do and never be afraid to be authentic.

Combing Through Chapter 3, Dread Locks

Rate your courage to express yourself on a scale of 1 to 10 (10 = no fear, and 1 = very fearful). Explore how and the way you ranked yourself.

How does your fear level affect your personal expressions (e.g., hair, clothing style, relationships)?

What's the most daring choice(s) you've made with your hair and appearance? Where were you when you did it? What made you take the risk?

Set a personal goal and timeline to "push the envelope" regarding your hair and beauty!

Jot down some kind words—or *hairlooms*—about your hair.

Diagram Your "Mane" Issue

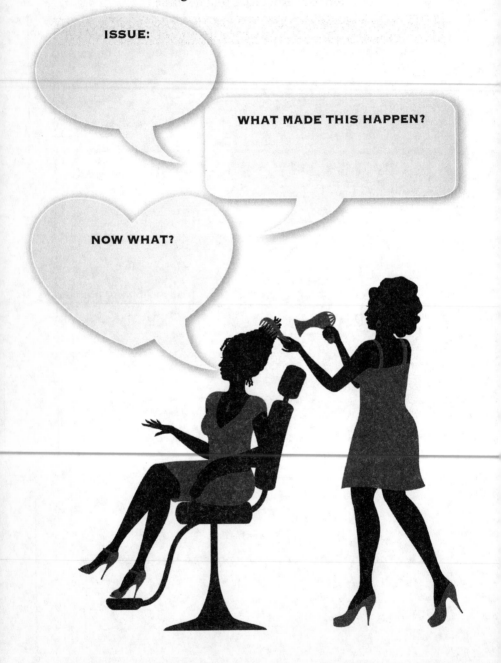

New Growth: Chart Your Solution

Now What?	What's the Effect?	What's Your Solution?
_____	_____	_____
_____	_____	_____
_____	_____	_____
_____	_____	_____
_____	_____	_____
_____	_____	_____
_____	_____	_____
_____	_____	_____
_____	_____	_____
_____	_____	_____
_____	_____	_____
_____	_____	_____
_____	_____	_____
_____	_____	_____

Chapter 4

THE MANE ATTRACTION

Millions gazed with wide-eyed wonder on Friday, April 29, 2011, as Prince William and Kate Middleton proclaimed their mutual, undying love. It appeared as if Kate's long, glossy, brunette tresses had wrapped themselves around her true-life Prince Charming's heart. No doubt her hair, and other traits, helped tie the love knot that would set the stage for a larger-than-life wedding. Amidst the nuptial splendor that was nothing short of a fairy tale, the newly appointed Duke and Duchess of Cambridge wed. The big event was high on the pecking order of story coverage for print and electronic news outfits, which had been covering the lead-up to the nuptials in excruciating detail. The world caught sneak peeks of the stunning British fascinators and succulent wedding desserts.

Broadcast coverage of the actual day revealed the brown, white, and beige faces of commoners and nobility. They pressed their way to catch a glimpse of the wedding that topped social media charts and made online history. The bride's sister, Pippa, had been living in relative obscurity before the wedding and suddenly became an overnight sensation. As the cameras panned the crowd of adoring fans on that historic day, it was common to see a wide array of expressions. Some could scarcely contain tears of joy. Other fans released peals of laughter and cheers with the force of well-orchestrated fireworks.

As people from India to Indiana were enraptured by this wedding, I made an observation. I found it curious that most of the excitement was expressed by women. As I began to casually ask different men about the event, several were dismissive and responded with a level of nonchalance: "Aren't you going to watch the Royal Wedding? I know you're not gonna miss it," I told a male coworker.

"For what?" he retorted. "If you've seen one wedding, you've seen 'em all. What's the big deal?" I couldn't just let this insensitive remark go unchallenged!

"You mean to tell me you will watch a regular old football game for hours and not the wedding? In case you forgot, *this* only happens once in a lifetime. You should at least show a little bit of excitement." Other male colleagues appeared equally annoyed by the amount of attention that this event was receiving. Some acted as if the royal wedding occurred regularly and deserved no more attention than paint drying on a kitchen wall.

Admittedly, their responses annoyed me, and I charged these men with numerous counts of insensitivity to marital love and off-the-charts testosterone levels. Before I forged ahead with my rant, a more objective conclusion crossed my mind. I considered the fact that the stage was set long ago for these divergent opinions.

Many women have spent their days creating "make believe" scenes in which they were the princesses and unwitting action figures or celebrities were the princes. I recall with pinpoint clarity the list of men who would seek my hand in marriage. As a five-year-old, I was making plans to marry Michael Jackson, David Cassidy, Robin (Batman's sidekick) and—last but not least—my kindergarten crush, Edwin. With no understanding of the concept of polygamy, I believed with every fiber of my imagination that I would marry the *men* of my dreams!

Now, I understand that all little girls don't find the same boys appealing. I believe, however, that there is a common cord that ties us together. Whether women envisioned a knight in shining armor sweeping them from a South Bronx stoop or whisking them away from a well-manicured lawn in Scarsdale, women everywhere can relate to a similar dream. Many women were raised on a steady diet of fairy tales that included beautiful maidens and chivalrous men whose only purpose in life was to rescue us. Subconsciously, they were taught to expect a "happily-ever-after" life. Simply put, they were raised to dream.

The challenge for many is that the dreams they have nurtured will not come true because they were built on the unstable foundation of wishful thinking. Women know all too well that life's storms have a way of crushing a foundation that was rooted in the pages of library books or the silver-screen images of the Saturday matinee. Reality has a way of sticking a pin in our proverbial bubble and clipping the wings of every fantasy. One solid dose of reality—at any age—is enough to make people abandon their visions of what life could be and should be for them.

While reality can cause women to neatly tuck dreams away, what storage vault can hold them indefinitely? They begin to pop out and wiggle their way into their lives. This truth is manifest as some women chase after the ghost man who is "the" prince. With an arm's-length list, women have charged into our stylized demographic with the hopes of finding one who has the right height, complexion, and temperament. Others find themselves believing that the dream is wrapped in expensive real estate and lavish lifestyles. The quest for a preferred brand of reality has become the true north and internal compass. For women, this truth could not be clearer than when it comes to their hair.

What little girl did not grow up dreaming of having long tresses that flowed in the wind? Each generation has its own hairstyle icon: Foxy Brown's perfectly shaped Afro, Shirley Temple's bouncing ringlets, and Farrah Fawcett's feathered coif. Hair has guided women like a beacon of light toward the apex of beauty since birth. Moms will clip a barrette with a bow on just a single strand of baby's hair to quickly distinguish Baby Jane from Baby Joe. The same locks are molded to perfection even as the shell of a woman is laid to rest in a coffin, the final touch-up before the curtain call on the stage of life.

Women of all races and ethnicities find themselves unwittingly occupied with hair and crestfallen when they fall short of public applause. Caucasian women may find themselves obsessing over the difficulty of finding the shampoo that will keep their hair manageable after its daily washing. Asian women may find themselves searching for the style or product that will make their straight tresses have more body. What African-American woman is not familiar with the quest for a product that will make her edges "lay down" until the next hair appointment? All women, to some degree, are caught in the tangle of hair's web.

Our early experiences shape us. What we see and hear has power. This principle applies to women's focus on hair. What better example of a first introduction to the power of hair than through fairy tales and animated movies? Storytellers throughout the centuries have introduced many giggly girls to the ideal that having the "right" hair is the gateway to splendor, riches, and romance.

The legendary story of "Goldilocks and the Three Bears" is yet another reminder of hair's prominence. We all know that these imaginary bears went for a walk as their porridge cooled, only to return to a house that had been invaded by none other than Goldilocks. While it is noteworthy to remember the fair maiden ate their porridge and broke their beds, for the purposes of our discussion, let's examine something else. It's interesting to note that this character's identifying characteristic is her hair. There is never a mention of Goldilocks' middle name or surname.

The comic strip-turned-Broadway hit, *Little Orphan Annie*, features a little girl who is best recognized by her mop of curly red hair. Even people who have never seen the play or read the comic strip can likely identify the character because of this.

Hair has never penned the world's greatest poetic stanzas or strummed melodies to soothe the aching soul. Yet people—women in particular—are attracted to hair on a level that even we are not able to fully comprehend. Media images have helped many women of color develop the idea that hair is important, but all hair is not equal. One look at my favorite television shows drove the point home. Since there were so few Black actors in the sixties and seventies, I personally idolized girls and women who looked nothing like me. Jan and Marcia Brady of *The Brady Bunch* and Laurie from *The Partridge Family* were my American idols. While two were blonde and one was a brunette, the common thread was their long, straight hair. As a child I believed, as most young children do, that life was a free-for-all—a fruit tree that had been planted on community property. The sweet and colorful delights hanging from the boughs were mine for the picking—I simply needed to find a way to reach up and grab them. My creativity was the key to finding the ladder that would take me where I needed to go.

Armed with the mental images of my television icons, I decided that I could make my hair look just like theirs. One look at my own tresses reminded me I was going to have to use a bit of ingenuity to live the dream. After all, my mother only allowed me to let my hair roam free on Easter Sunday and perhaps on Children's Day at church. Outside these annual events, my hair was neatly controlled in a braided style. When I did wear my hair in an open style, it was puffier than theirs and shorter. The texture also made it impossible for my tresses to swing and bounce.

I would need to find something to give my hair the desired movement. I searched for an object in our New York City apartment that would do the trick. Finally, I came across a clean, white cloth diaper. I placed it on my head, adjusting the position, until it covered my hair and dangled over my shoulders and down my back. I secured my "locs" in place with some of my mother's bobby pins and shook my head back and forth, readjusting the pins until I was sure the diaper wouldn't fall off. My final challenge was to make my "hair" blow in the wind like that of my TV idols. The kind of wind I needed for flowing tresses was not blowing across 167th Street between Findley and Teller Avenues in the South Bronx.

Undaunted by this minor hiccup in my beauty plan, I found the wind I needed by plugging in a metal three-speed fan. As I stood directly in front it, my flowing cloth diaper whipped around my head. I shook it violently from side to side and prayed that my "hair" would not get caught in the metal blades. For a few precious moments, I felt as if I finally measured up to the images I'd seen on television. It's amazing how quickly women and girls can buy into the ill-conceived belief that resembling a television icon is a recipe for acceptance. They often agree to live with poet Samuel Taylor Coleridge's "willing suspension of disbelief." On a cerebral level, they know that they look nothing like the actresses they admire on the screen. On an emotional level, though, some Black women unconsciously desire the look of the primetime images that dart across the TV and movie screens. The majority of these icons are Caucasian women with a glam squad available to polish their physical features as needed. We forget the fact that coily kinky hair, darker skin, and full noses are physical traits rarely noted as standards of beauty in Hollywood and other forms of media. We forget that often, the look we seek is not the look that is inherently ours.

Where are attractions born? Often, it's hard to determine what tickles our senses to the point of surrender. Perhaps it's a scent—the smell of a certain aftershave attracts you to a man because it's the kind your beloved dad wore, and it reminds you of him. It could be something you've seen before—an expensive suit in a store window reminds you of the take-charge business executive you saw at a conference, so you buy it hoping to have the same impact. We all fall prey to intangibles that are the fuel for attractions.

It's those subconscious, suggestive nudges that make us pick up the decadent, high-calorie dessert even though we swear we need to lose weight. While we may, indeed, know what drives us to have our senses satisfied, it is a bit more difficult to understand how these gentle pulls entered our worlds. While some attractions are good—love at first sight might lead to a long and happy marriage—some might lead us down a path of danger and into a lifetime of regret. Growing up in a dysfunctional home, for instance, might make a woman recreate the unhealthy family dynamic ingrained in her from decades past. When we become shackled to the attraction, our affinities can leave us imprisoned in some way.

An explanation of magnetism helps us to understand why we readily accept or reject the things and people to whom we are introduced. Insight into this phenomenon is particularly helpful for Black women as we honestly examine our draw to certain standards of beauty and a rejection of others. Whether you attended public or private schools, it's safe to say that most elementary school lessons included a class on magnetic attraction. The hands-on, demonstrated lesson about magnetic attraction fit the bill for the kids, who naturally hated lectures. While I might have gone glassy-eyed over discussions of the periodic table of elements, I grew wide-eyed and eager when I was offered an opportunity to see silver-and-red horseshoe magnets defy the mighty, invisible force field. I was fascinated by the magnetic power that mysteriously shifted clumps of fine lead shavings across a piece of paper.

What kept some magnets from touching, even in the face of applied force? What made the lead shavings passively follow the push of the magnet? The same properties govern human relationship dynamics, and we can find the answers to these questions by taking a closer look in this direction. A casual inventory of the people who fit into the confines of our inner circle likely reveals that opposites indeed attract.

Let's look at one of the basic ways that men and women are different—aside from anatomy. Studies report that women speak an

average of 20,000 words per day in comparison to their male coun-
terparts, who only utter 7,000 words daily.[1] Based on these stats, I am
all woman! I wake up and go to sleep with words, thoughts, and jokes
spewing from my mouth. I've even been told that even sleep doesn't
muzzle me; sources say I continue to talk when not fully conscious!
Kyle, my husband, is the epitome of a man of few words. After nine
years of marriage, I've come to realize that the differences in our com-
munication styles actually drew me to him. I'm intrigued by the fact
that he can share so little and yet say so much. I'm captivated by the
way his silence speaks and answers questions without uttering a single
word. I am magnetized by my husband because, in many ways, he is
nothing like me.

In stark contrast to Kyle's quiet nature, I am embarrassed to say
that people who are naturally "motor mouths" irk me to no end. I
can't get a complete thought out before my words face the chopping
block of their impulsive need to insert a clever story or phrase. Like
eager horses at the racetrack gate, they share multiple talking points
and illustrations of the previous points they've just shared. While
moments with incessant talkers can zap my energy and make me give
the side-eye, in truth, they are more like me than not. As we shift our
attention to the issue of what magnetizes Black women, these illustrations are completely applicable. As quiet as it's kept, many Black
women and girls operate by the "opposites attract" principle. This
attraction to opposites starts at an early age.

The historic 1940s "doll experiment" disclosed that 63 percent of
Black girls who were polled preferred playing with White dolls versus
Black dolls.[2] Recent attempts at this experiment cite slight changes
in little Black girls' preferences, but nothing significant. The genetic
makeup of Black women dictates that our skin will generally be a

shade of brown, and our hair will feature kinks or coils. The overwhelming push to get our hair and skin to look vastly different than it naturally does speaks volumes. Aside from those who straighten for convenience or legitimate blemishes, the attraction to a "look" that is acutely distinct from our natural attributes is telling.

Beneath the shroud of social poise and presentation, the law of magnetism is operating. Two north poles and two south poles—regardless of human effort—will never come together. These poles remain forever separated by the force of magnetic repulsion. At the core, some Black women feel a hidden aversion to anything resembling themselves. This firmly planted disdain for their style of beauty has taken root because of unkind or careless words spoken about their hair.

This truth explains the importance women place on hair and beauty. It starts when we are youngsters, where there is an unwritten but widely known standard about which hair textures and skin shades are more favorable in the family. Black girls approaching adolescence may have brushed down baby hairs or tried their hand at a Jheri curl hoping to catch the cute guy. When they reach young adulthood, some Black women have a standing appointment at the beauty salon for chemical treatments every four to six weeks to make sure that their tresses are acceptable in corporate settings. What bride has not, did not, or will not spend hours poring over beauty magazines? She is hopeful that she will find the hairstyle that will be the envy of every woman on her wedding day.

My sister is a doctor, and over the sleep-deprived years of study it takes to become one, she collected textbooks—lots of them. She had a bookcase loaded with volumes of writings from her undergraduate and medical school studies. By all accounts, the bookcase should have been able to handle the weight of these texts, but, much to my sister's shock, the bookshelf collapsed at the most inopportune time, sending books tumbling to the floor and causing a mini-earthquake. The piece of furniture was simply not strong enough to carry the weight of so many books that were collectively so heavy.

While we likely don't admit it, hair has become the shelf upon which we both wittingly and unwittingly rest the volumes of our lives. From our childhood to adulthood, we subconsciously collect these experiences, comments, and actions and put them into heavy volumes that we tote around for the rest of our lives. These are the emotional weights; they are too heavy for us to bear, so we shift onto our hair. As with my sister's bookcase, our hair was never designed to handle the pressure. Its primary function is to protect the body, but we've made it an adornment. Hair—by definition—was never meant to define who we were, are, and will be. When this attraction is misplaced, our self-image begins to collapse beneath the weight of a lie, and we are wounded.

One weekend while in North Carolina with family, a Caucasian lady approached me and said she was attracted to my natural hairstyle. "Wow! Isn't your hair the cutest. I love your curls." This complete stranger went on to say, "I wish my hair was like yours. I always wear my hair the same way all the time."

In disbelief that she would never switch it up, I responded, "I'm sure you can wear some different styles. You should try it. You never know; you may look cuter than you think!"

We began to talk about the challenges of styling our hair. As we ended the conversation, this woman briefly told me something that shocked me.

"I would stop wearing the same old ponytail, but it covers up my wound. I was shot in the head." This woman nonchalantly and boldly pointed to her bullet wound, but I could barely see it. The bullet wound had been strategically covered by her choice of hairstyle, but the hole was still there.

The encounter with this woman shows me that she is not the only one who uses hair to cover an area that has been wounded and remains tender to the touch. Black women have been fed multiple servings of public opinion that deny any inherent beauty, delicacy, or physical acceptability. Left untreated, there is a tendency for women to become magnetized by what has been deemed beautiful and dismiss styles that are indigenous to whom they are. As appealing as twists, braids, or locs may be, some Black women will never wear them. The wound they may have experienced has handcuffed them to a past that, in all actuality, is a painful memory. Honest reflections may cause them to admit that they have placed their hair expressions under house arrest. Their tresses never receive a pass for good behavior because someone told them that their hair was bad.

While I was shocked that the woman I met in North Carolina had been grazed in the head by a bullet, and somewhat taken aback by her nonchalant discussion of it in terms of hairstyling issues, the reality is that her ponytail was blond and always acceptable.

The issue of acceptance has been an undercurrent in my life and other Black women's lives from the cradle to the grave. I have seen the grieving break the pace of plans to lay the dearly departed to rest for a hair appointment. I have known patients in hospital beds who writhed in pain yet mustered the strength to make sure their hair was in place before undergoing surgery. Personal historical accounts readily reveal that hair truly has its own limitations. It is no rival for twisted images and vestiges of ravaged self-worth. Hair can cover the head, but it is woefully unable to cover the heart.

The mane attraction has affected many areas of Black women's lives, but this force does not have to reign from a seat of authority. The pull of polarity is not weakened with mere hands. Its force field is not penetrated by the lance or laser. The power of hair's magnetism is brought to its knees by an inside job.

A popular and clever credit-card television ad campaign has entertained us with creative monologues from a celebrity pitchman, which then ends with the iconic slogan, "What's in your wallet?" We all know that this question should be posed when assessing interest rate accrual and daily purchases. Additionally, we should know what objects in our wallets or pocketbooks are responsible for corrupting our debit and credit card's magnetic stripe.

If you've ever had your card demagnetize—usually because it's scratched or rendered useless by your cell phone—you know how frustrating and annoying it can be. Numerous swipes and heated rants do nothing to restore the now-destroyed magnetic field. In the wake of this aftermath, we scramble to find another card at the point of purchase and then need to remember to get a new card, which can be time-consuming and just add more to our long to-do list. Before pointing an accusing finger at some computer geek's stealthy attempt at identity theft, we need to understand that something we possessed actually destroyed the magnetism.

Likewise, it's important that Black women understand that their worth is not wrapped around rollers and rod-sets. The best of who we are is never purchased at the counter of a high-end salon. An attraction to hair needs to be recognized for what it is. This uncontrollable lure to hair does not define our best self. Denying this fact leads us to the lie that we have embraced our true identity just because we decided to "go natural." This faulty thinking may engender a sense of entitlement that grants us a pass for despising and demeaning women whose hair and features are the polar opposite of those of a typical Black woman.

Our goal should be an attraction to the inner qualities that uniquely mark us. A steely resolve to embrace our personalities, characters, and flaws will help us place hair and beauty in their proper places. This renewed perspective is the key that corrupts a flawed magnetic field of attraction. Like a literal key, it is generally kept close to our person. When Black women allow themselves be captivated by the warm sway of their inner beauty, the war of attraction is no longer waged. The "mane attraction" is replaced by the "me attraction." We are then candidates for hair *peace*.

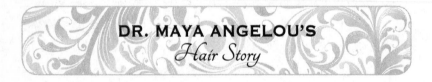

DR. MAYA ANGELOU'S
Hair Story

DR. MAYA ANGELOU *was a prolific, highly decorated author and poet. She received thirty honorary degrees and was the former Reynolds Professor of American Studies at Wake Forest University. A recipient of the Presidential Medal of Arts in 2000, she also received the National Medal of Arts in that same year. Noted for her autobiographical* I Know Why the Caged Bird Sings *(Random House), Dr. Angelou also wrote the poem "Amazing Peace" for President George W. Bush and delivered the poem at the 2005 national Christmas tree lighting ceremony. President Barack Obama presented Dr. Angelou with the Presidential Medal of Freedom, the country's highest civilian honor, in 2010.*

I have always liked I how look. It's my blessing. In my family, everyone was pleased with everyone's hair. My personal hair story invokes laughter, mostly.

I am told that many women have been influenced by my hair. In about 1952, I had received a scholarship to study dance in New York City. My son was seven years old, and I was twenty-four. I took him to New York and studied with Pearl Primus.* I worked at Metropolitan Life Insurance while I worked with Miss Primus. She was about 5'6" and she seemed to float. Oh, she was incredible. She taught African dance, and we sweated so much that my hair became very curly. So when I came to New York, I found a beautician; within two or three days, though, my hair was springing again.

Miss Primus had her hair cut, and I eventually had my hair cut into a short Afro. Some years later—Odetta the singer** and Abbey Lincoln*** and Miriam Makeba****—we all had our hair cut. And when I returned to San Francisco, my mother and brother—whose hair was straight with a wave in it—said that they loved my hair. But a man in the street saw me and said, "Aren't you Vivian and Clidell's daughter?" I said, "Yes Sir." He gave me $5 and said, "Go get something done to your head!"

In 1960 I had been in Europe with *Porgy and Bess*, and I came back in a ship from Naples, Italy, to New York City. A steward took me to my room, and there was another bed in the room. She said, "You will have an older woman as a roommate." I was so tired that I sat on the side of the bed—I had on slacks—and I fell asleep. About an hour later, I heard the steward speaking in Italian and saying to my roommate, "There is another woman in here, and she's lying down. Try not to disturb her." So the steward went out and the roommate came close to my bed. I pulled the drape back and sat up. My roommate screamed in Italian and went running. "There's a Black man in my room. There's a Black man in my room (*C'è un uomo nero nella mia stanza)!*" The steward came back and said, "That is not a Black man; it's a woman!" My roommate called another older lady to come to the room.

These two women—because of my hair—presumed I was a man. When they found I was a woman, they looked after me because of my hair difficulty!

The woman who knows that the first impression is a lasting one is intelligent. What people see first are those features that stand out, and for the African-American woman, the hair stands out because it frames the face. So you can have the prettiest face and no frame and, alas, your face does not get the attention you want. I think this is why women dye their hair blond, dark, and brunette—because they are aware of their first appearances. African-American women—whether we wear braids, cornrows, Jheri curls, perms, or big 'Fros—are usually meticulous about our hair. In some cases, we usually go to the same beautician until she dies or you do.

I would encourage the next generation to know that their features are gifts given by the Creator. Stay clean! See your body as it is—God-made and wonderfully wrought. It's amazing what presenting a clean face to the mirror will do for you in the morning. It's amazing what a clean body does for you. When you decide you want to put on makeup, put it on a clean face. You decide you're going to use perfume, put it on a clean body. You'll be amazed at how much you like yourself. If you want to dye your hair green because you want it green, that's what you should do. If you want to have your nose fixed because you want it fixed—not because it's the trend—do it.

Pearl Primus was a contemporary of Katherine Dunham, who had one of the most successful dance careers in American and European theater of the twentieth century and has been called the "Matriarch and Queen Mother of Black Dance." (November 29, 1919—October 29, 1994)

**Odetta was an American singer, actress, and songwriter. This civil and human rights activist has been heralded as "The Voice of the Civil Rights Movement." (December 31, 1930–December 2, 2008)*

***Abbey Lincoln was a civil rights activist. Also a jazz vocalist, she wrote and performed her own compositions. (August 6, 1930–August 14, 2010)*

****Miriam Makeba was a South African singer and activist. She fought against the South African system of apartheid. (March 4, 1932–November 9, 2008)*

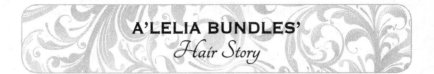

A'LELIA BUNDLES'
Hair Story

A'LELIA BUNDLES *is the great-great granddaughter of the first Black female millionaire and hair care creator Madam C. J. Walker. A seasoned journalist and public speaker, she has also authored the* New York Times *bestseller,* On Her Own Ground: The Life and Times of Madam C. J. Walker *(Scribner). A'Lelia has partnered with Sundial Brands (Shea Moisture) to create the Madam C. J. Walker Beauty Culture hair care products, which are distributed through Sephora stores nationwide.*

Now, I probably had more specific anxiety and angst about deciding to go natural than the average person. The politics were playing themselves out in my household in a way that probably didn't happen in most people's households. When I was twelve and getting ready to take swimming lessons, I got a perm. I had long hair, and we figured that would be easier. So at that stage—it was 1964—getting a perm was a normal thing to do. My dad, at that point, was president of Summit Laboratories, which was a company that made a product called Hair Straight. It was one of the main Black-owned hair care companies that had developed in the fifties.

In 1969, when I was a senior in high school, Afros were really very popular. At that age, I was a very politically aware person, and I really wanted an Afro. This may seem like an irony to a lot of people because of their misconceptions of Madam Walker and their belief that she invented the hot comb. I was becoming very conscious of being Black and the symbolism of being Black in that era. Unique to other people's households, we had hair wars in my house because my father was very much opposed to me getting an Afro because his company made hair straighteners. My mother

Hairlooms

thought differently. She said, "Hair is hair. You have to use shampoo and conditioner whether you have a perm or not."

Nonetheless, my mother took me down to the Walker Beauty School, and I left with this really huge Afro hairstyle. I wore an Afro until the end of college and cut it very short by my senior year. For the next two decades, I really went back and forth between short hair, long hair, and permed hair. I got to the point—in my late thirties or so—where I just didn't like the way my hair felt when it was permed. It felt like straw to me. At that time, I was wearing it long and going to the beauty shop every two weeks to get it styled and sit under the dryer. I would go to my hair dresser at 8:00 in the morning before I went to work. One day I went, and the stylist didn't show up. At that point, I said, "Forget this. I'm cutting my hair!"

For the last twenty years, I've worn my hair short and natural. I just prefer doing it that way because I don't really want to spend time on it. I'm too busy. I've got too many other things that are more important to me than doing my hair. Having said this about me personally, I love it when I see all of these great permed or natural styles.

We—as African-American women—need to love ourselves. We can still have permed hair and love ourselves. We don't need to feel like we are doing this because we have to. Ironically, to me, I've had a lot of young women tell me that they can't get a job on Wall Street or a job at a law firm if they wear their hair natural. This thought is just not true, but people have let it become ingrained in their minds. There is a certain professional way you can wear your hair natural. Realistically speaking, there are probably certain styles you can't have—straight or natural—in a corporate environment. I have too many friends who are very successful as attorneys or businesswomen who have natural hair. I know that you can do it.

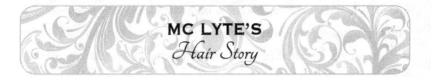

MC LYTE'S *Hair Story*

MC LYTE *is a legendary rapper and recording artist, and the first African-American woman to be named president of the Los Angeles Chapter of the Grammy Recording Academy.*

I remember a time when I got my hair cut into what I thought was a style. I had someone cut it, and the new style was very shocking for me. After getting that hairdo, I deliberately kept it wet and curly for about eleven or twelve months. I wanted to give my hair some time to grow again. This new look was a detriment to me at the time that it happened. I had already released a record that was successful. I had already created a look for myself. With this new cut, I looked really different, and the public had grown accustomed to seeing me look a certain way. To make up for the difference, I wore a headband to make my in-between phase less obvious. Nobody ever saw the magnitude of the cut at all! There are pictures of me—I think in 1985—with the little head wrap that I was wearing around it, and only the top of my head was exposed.

After this experience, I realized that hair changes can affect artists much more than the audience. I think the audience is open to the idea of artists making changes. I think the audience wants me to do new and creative things with my appearance. While they like new looks, I don't think fans want changes that make their favorite artist look unrecognizable. When this happens, it's hard for the audience to relate to the artist.

Over time, I also realized that a hairstyle that works for somebody else may not work for you. It took me a really long time to see that straight hair is not for me, because I was around a lot of people who wore their hair straight. I'm not saying that I won't wear it straight again, because I never want to put myself in that box. Since my hair is natural, though, I found I'm more free when I wear my hair curly versus straight. I can go to the gym when I want to. I can go to the beach, or I can go to the pool. It can rain, and I'm not having a heart attack. There is just a level of freedom that comes along with wearing my hair curly. You have to be ready for that level of freedom, as well. For the young ladies coming up, I think it's important for them to understand who they really are. I encourage them to wear different styles and try it all! When I look back on all of the changes I have made with my hairstyles, I realize that hair is just hair. I think that sometimes we make it too huge.

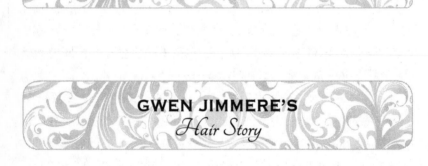

GWEN JIMMERE'S
Hair Story

GWEN JIMMERE *is the first Black woman to hold a patent for a natural hair care product. As the founder and CEO of, Naturalicious, she has grown her beauty industry startup into one of the fastest-growing hair care companies in the United States. Naturalicious is the first company to develop an all-natural, patented hair care system that does the work of thirteen products in only four simple steps and is proven and guaranteed to take you from wash to style in less than an hour. The line is sold in select Whole Foods stores, all Mustard Seed Market locations, and other fine retailers and boutiques across the United States, Indonesia, and Trinidad.*

Naturalicious was named one of the top six beauty brands in the United States by Black Enterprise *magazine and was the only beauty brand invited to participate in President Obama's Inaugural Ball, where Gwen had the honor of including her entire suite of products in all VIP gift bags. Gwen has also been featured in the* Washington Post *and* Essence *magazine.*

I went natural because I was pregnant with my son. I had no intentions of staying natural. I had planned to be natural just for the nine-month period. I knew that anything you put on your body has a very good chance of getting into your bloodstream. If you're pregnant, that can affect your child. So at that time, I was relaxing my hair. The minute I realized I was pregnant, though, I made the decision. I noticed that when I wasn't using a relaxer, my hair got so much thicker, longer, and fuller. It wasn't breaking or nearly as scraggly. It was amazing! So even after my son was born, I decided to continue the natural hair journey. So I should thank him for putting me on this path to loving my beauty as I was created.

When I used a relaxer, I hated my hair. If you had told me in high school that I'd end up loving my hair, I would have laughed at you. In retrospect, the way I felt about my hair was how I felt about my beauty. I always thought I was pretty but still felt that I could be better. I think that how you feel about your hair is an extension of how you feel about yourself. Most people don't realize that. How you feel about yourself extends to so many different things in life. It extends to career choices. It extends to things you accept in relationships as you get older. It extends to how you raise your children.

My choice also affected other areas of my life. Over time, I realized that I was becoming very deliberate and intentional about the products and ingredients I put in my hair. I started to wonder what would happen if I had that same intention about the foods I put into my body. Being natural with my hair has caused me to be more conscious about the food that I eat.

I started to pay attention to the quality of food that I ate and how it affected me. I eventually noticed that I had so much energy! Now I can keep up with my son because I'm eating more quality food. All of these changes were based on my hair decision.

It's very important to embrace what we have. Most people don't like what they have because they don't know what to do with it. Once you find out how to make it work, then you become more appreciative of what you have. God makes no mistakes. If He wanted us to have straight hair, we would have had it. If He wanted us to have blue eyes, we would have had them. We were created to be beautiful. We should find out what to do with our beauty so we can appreciate it.

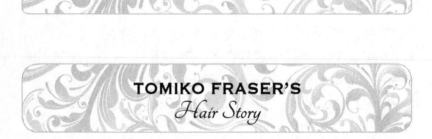

TOMIKO FRASER'S
Hair Story

TOMIKO FRASER *is the first African-American woman signed by Maybelline to an exclusive contract. Her impressive eight-year stint with Maybelline makes her the longest-serving spokesperson for any cosmetics company. Countless billboards, magazine ads, and commercials on behalf of the cosmetics brand have featured Tomiko. These include Tommy Hilfiger, Alfani, The Gap, Old Navy, Lee Jeans, and Target, and she has graced the pages of magazines around the world, including German* Vogue, Glamour, *British* Marie Claire, Cosmopolitan, Essence, *and* Elle. *In 2016, she landed a spot in the global commercial for Lancôme's signature fragrance, La Vie Est Belle.*

Years ago, I developed a sensitivity to relaxers. My hair would break off whenever I put relaxers in it, and a scalp specialist told me I needed to stop using them altogether. I was mortified, and I would wear tracks or a weave to cover it up. I still have two big bins of wigs in my closet that I haven't worn for years. When I got them, I thought I had to have hair to be sexy.

As my hair began to become healthy, I decided to give it a chance. In time, I decided to wear my hair in its natural state. I had really been drawn to women—even those who I saw on TV—who had cut off their hair. I just found that look really attractive. I consulted with my husband, and he said, "As long as you're happy, I'm happy." My most powerful, freeing, childlike moment was when I chose for myself and cut it off. I didn't ask my agent or even tell him, initially. That was the moment when I did my "big chop."

Now, you can't tell me I'm not cute with my natural hair! I won't even stay in the room for the conversation. I always thought that I had to have long hair to be sexy, but now you can't tell me I'm not sexy. I'm not conceited, but I have confidence. I finally got it because I decided I was going to determine what was beautiful for me. It has just been amazing. I don't push people to go natural or wear a weave. I just personally think you should be confident in whatever you choose to wear.

Across the board, I would say that we should *self-define* our beauty. I understand that we have societal, religious, and traditional expectations. Take those things off your neck and *do you*. If that means you want to shave off some of your hair and wear a green dress with purple shoes, then go ahead. Hair grows back, so try different things. Keep trying until you find the *you* that you know you are. When it comes to hair, you may not know what your style is right away.

Over the many centuries, longer hair has been thought of as more beautiful. I think this idea has just put pressure on women to wear their hair in a certain way. I have many non-Black friends who have complained about not having the hair they want. Some want it curly, straight, or short. For years, I have heard my friends of different ethnicities talk about their hair in one way or the other; they wanted highlights or had an issue with split ends. They don't seem to like the hair that comes out of their heads.

In general, we as women tend to be harsh with ourselves. Inside, though, we are just little girls. I think that if we didn't talk down to ourselves and instead started to be kind, loving feelings about ourselves would eventually start to stick. So when we have those moments when we're not completely in love with ourselves, we should see the little girl in the mirror and encourage her to be in love with herself. It may not happen at once, but start with your hair and get to the point where you love the bottoms of your feet. The hair is the first thing that people see on you, and they make a judgment based on that. If you can embrace your hair, you can embrace your eyes or hips, and embrace your thighs. You have to start somewhere.

Combing Through Chapter 4,
The Mane Attraction

Fill in the blank: I am attracted to hair that is _____.
Explain your answer. _____
_____
_____

Describe a time when you hid behind an outward attribute (e.g., intelligence, appearance, accomplishments). What pushed you to that point? Was it a good *cover*?
_____
_____
_____

A Japanese proverb states that, "The nail that sticks out gets hammered down." How comfortable are you "sticking out" when it comes to your hair and appearance? Rate yourself on a scale of 1–10 (10 = very comfortable, and 1 = very uncomfortable).
_____
_____
_____

Which of your inner qualities are most attractive to you?
_____
_____
_____

Jot down some kind words—or *hairlooms*—about your hair.
_____
_____

Diagram Your "Mane" Issue

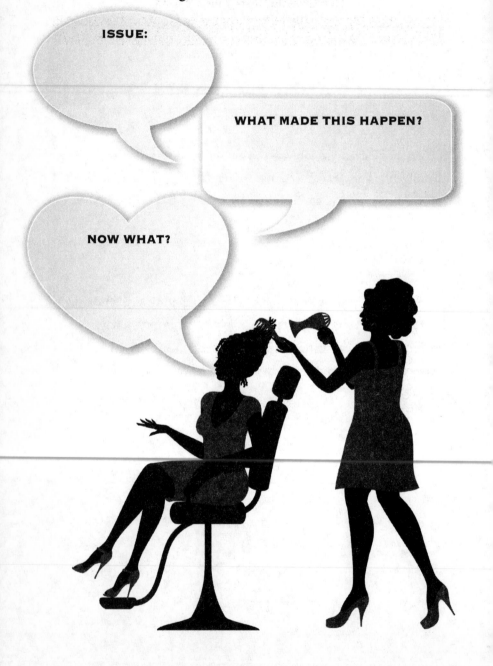

New Growth: Chart Your Solution		
Now What?	What's the Effect?	What's Your Solution?

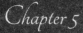

Chapter 5

HAIR PEACE

N ot one for rules, I circular-filed the "dark girls shouldn't wear bright colors" memo years ago. As a mocha-skinned, pudgy preschooler, I refused to sport drab colors to New York City's iconic Coney Island. There was no way I was going to get on the Magic Carpet and other kiddie rides unless I was wearing my sunny yellow and white polka-dot halter dress. On that day, my dress was brighter than the mustard that I slathered across my Nathan's hot dog. My juried classical piano performance and fire-engine red chiffon dress were crowd favorites during my tween years. When I was eighteen, I just knew that a bright color was a must for the first annual Harlem Week activities, so I wore my bright orange peplum dress—a chart-topper on that Sunday in August 1984. After all, this event was my official "Goodbye Tour" before trading my jet-set Big Apple life for a quiet, calm college life in pastoral central Pennsylvania.

Hours of rotary-dial phone chatter with my teenage mod squad suggested that I wear this super-cute orange masterpiece. I'm sure the sun blushed a bit with one glimpse of the hug that this tropical dress put my developing curves. A signature cheesy grin framed my face and added the personal stamp for my pick. The flounce on this dress showcased my ankle-strapped, brown leather sandals. Several gold-tone bracelets gave my outfit the final polish it needed to hit the festival in grand style. Each homemade curlicue bounced along the steamy Harlem streets. A sign of the times, I had someone take a photo of me in my sunny ensemble with the now-vintage 110 camera.

Weeks later—once in my freshman college dorm—I taped this photo to the inside flap of my cloth-covered diary. Still there more than thirty years later, the adhesive has since dried, but the image is cemented in my mind. I recall instances when I would peek at this photo while sitting on my twin-sized dorm bed. Instantly, my orange image transported me to the warmth of that day. This dash of color winked and waved at me during the "freshman fifteen," all-night cram sessions, and budding forever friendships. Orange became the warmth that blanketed one of my fondest memories. Orange was my color.

The ray of a shining moment, no matter how bright, can be eclipsed by the shroud of life-altering events. Some periods in life can land a blow that causes flashbacks to reel. Hit hard enough, these blows with new realities can wring pleasant moments dry and drain them of their once-vibrant colors.

My moment came twenty-three years later.

This particular August memory carried none of the Harlem Week's dazzle. Indeed, the color orange made its appearance again, but this time I barely knew the person who wore it. My chillingly awkward encounter with him was now on display for a hand-selected jury and judge to examine. I remember seeing the ill-fitted, orange prison uniform cover his husky frame. The gold-tone bangles that I remember were replaced with stainless steel handcuffs in plain view. His ankles were not strapped with leather sandals, but ankle cuffs that made his steps measured and calculated.

Come on, Michele. Hang in there; the worst is almost over, I told myself. Heart-pounding fear had turned my best intentions to vapor; my hands felt like ice. I stroked my chilly palms in an act of self-soothing, but the rest of my body was motionless. *How long is this trial going to take? I want to leave now,* I thought. Always one for eye contact, that day I just couldn't look at his face. My head hung limp, but my neck had just enough strength to lift my eyes into the stares of an anonymous crowd that would eventually decide his fate. *I just can't look him in the eye. I know it's stupid,* I mentally chided myself, *but I feel like he'll know what I'm thinking. He'll know I'm scared. I can't cry now.* Random spots in the courtroom became my constant focus as my mind raced. My mind ran past questions that demanded answers: *What if he breaks out of the shackles? Is he really going to jail? Will he sexually assault me again?*

Unanswerable questions can be a cruel taskmaster. If allowed into your head, they can steal sleep from your eyes and leave you in a stupor by daybreak. A few years later, I do have some answers to some questions. I know his name. I know his age. I know his motive. There are other questions, however, that I likely will never know. As the years have rolled along, I've had to place a "hard return" so that my life would not resemble a run-on sentence with no apparent end. Instinctively, I knew that turning the heavy pages of the sexual assault would only be possible if I returned. I really needed to backtrack to the spot. I wanted to revisit the actual place of the attack a few months later.

Standing alone outside the bank, I began to reconcile the images I remembered against what I actually saw that fateful evening. Now in broad daylight, I thought, *Boy, does this place look different.* Like a photographer, I checked my punch list of mental images. *This is where I stood barefoot in the grass after fighting him off; I was so out of breath. Those jeans were my favorites, but I won't be wearing those again.* I turned my head and thought, *Yep. That's the curb where the police car pulled up. And that's the glass door I pushed through. This is the spot where it all happened.*

A little braver and bolder, I casually inched toward the enclosed ATM. My then-makeshift boxing ring appeared much smaller than I recalled. I was ready to make a new transaction as my once-shaky hands now brushed across the ATM keypad with deliberate strokes. This time, I didn't need to reposition disheveled hairs; there were no shallow breaths to take. This time, I began to control my response to the trauma. This time, I chose to see the attack in the light of day.

You can always tell when the healing balm of time has paid your ransom. My decision to patronize the bank where the attack occurred was a sign. I also knew I was making peace with my storied past when I gave orange another place in my wardrobe. I did not avoid or bypass these landmark events to make peace with my love for the color orange. I found my place of calm by realistically allowing them to exist in my memory bank. While on opposite ends of life's color spectrum, both are associated with orange. Both are associated with me.

Life is filled with polarities. This experience taught me that good days and bad days don't have to "duke it out" to gain peace. Peace does not kick out either event, but invites them both to stay. Each, however, is then assigned boundaries and a specific room in my mind.

As Black women comb through—on different levels—the challenge of accepting our natural hair and beauty, the question arises: "How can we achieve peace with what we've been given at birth?" The answer comes as we define peace. Peace is not the absence of conflicting images, thoughts, and conclusions. On the contrary, the peaceful understand and accept that life's pages are filled with "and" rather than "or." We have joy *and* sorrow. We know terror *and* triumph. The peaceful eventually allows both to coexist. It is the prized emotional state that is nimble enough to embrace the fact that pleasantries and pain both exist. People absolutely love and completely hate—concurrently—the same person, idea, food, and artistic expression. The same proverbial glass is viewed as half-empty and half-full. For me, orange signifies the worst in others, *and* orange signified the best in me. I chose to bend toward the latter even though I accept the former.

My struggle for self-acceptance really has been with embracing the acceptable and unacceptable things I received at birth. My creativity easily lent itself to fantasy. However, serious movement toward peace really called for me to squarely look some truths in the eye and settle them once and for all.

My mother shared a comment that one of my aunts made about me when I was about two months old. This relative was not awestruck by my budding signs of giftedness or ability to carry the family-line name, Pecolia. Instead, my mother tells me that this aunt stated the obvious: Michele has big thighs! Now, mind you, after a few months in the world, we don't resemble what we'll look like after an infusion of hormones and carbs. Some things are bound for change, and others will remain. For instance, my mom says I was fair-skinned at birth; a few weeks later, however, my skin shaded to dark brown. Nearly bald for my first couple of years, my hair eventually crawled from my scalp to the nape of my neck. My thighs? They are another story. Call it prescience or detection, but my aunt was completely accurate. These beauties were, are, and will always be the most ample part of my body. The only way for them to comfortably fit into my pencil skirts and skinny jeans is to turbo-charge my gym workouts. Peace came as I framed my thoughts about myself in reality. My thighs can always be more trim, but they will never be slim. Why? Because they weren't small when I came out of the womb!

Black women can begin to make peace by accepting that certain tensions exist and making a personal choice about the one to which they will cling. Choices will always be the paint that creates pictures of peace upon the canvas of life. A decision to silence the squawk of toxic thoughts about your hair makes way for tranquility. The resolve to personally affirm your unique beauty—despite public opinions— ushers in "calm" to its reserved seat in your emotions. Choice gives the nod for peace to storm through confusion and balance the scales of the heart. When we face ourselves and choose to pursue peace, we become empowered. The Earth's crust may not move, but the ground on which we stand will begin to settle. This choice empowers us to applaud our performance when there are still remaining movements in the acts of our lives. When we are at peace with ourselves, we quickly upstage our understudy. We proudly take the spotlight and refuse to hide behind the curtain that hides our true identity.

Achieving this measure of contentedness is not quick and can easily be mistaken. It takes a self-aware, discerning eye to accurately judge whether we're okay with ourselves. The absence of peace is always present in noticeable ways. We may wear our hair in its natural state, but the incessant internal upheaval and instability still plagues us. Nocturnal tosses and endless hunts for the cool side of the proverbial pillow are signs that we are not at rest. Just because we're natural doesn't mean we have peace. Faulty metrics can easily fool the unsuspecting and make us think we have reached a destination when, in essence, we're still on a journey.

For years, money was my barometer for self-acceptance. After all, what real Black woman wouldn't make a financial investment in her appearance? I knew firsthand about the cost of transitioning from my mother's kitchen to a beauty parlor to get my hair washed and pressed. The shiny curls were always attached to a price tag. On many occasions, I had to scrape change together for my four-to-six-week perm "fix" during my college and grad school years. Low-income times meant having a DIY experience with a drugstore perm and friend-turned-stylist. Any discomfort that I had about the way my hair responded throughout the years was placed at bay with product purchases. I was a sucker for a product's promise that my hair that would defy its genetic composition and stay straight when wet. I can't tell you the thousands of dollars I spent trying to achieve hair acceptance. Unwanted jars, tubes, and bottles of hair potions told the story. As my bank account ached to stay full, my need for hair acceptance caused me to be overdrawn in more ways than one. I hate to say it, but there were even times I wouldn't pay utilities and rent on time because it was "essential" that I paid to get my hair done. I justified my spending habits because the price really defined my acceptance of how I looked.

Or did it?

The quest for the best price always makes me think about the popular television game show, *The Price Is Right*. Scores of screaming contestants prepare to run down the studio aisle when the announcer says, "Come on down, you're the next contestant on *The Price Is Right!*"

As quiet as it's kept, I have lived vicariously through these TV strangers. My stomach has felt the mounting anxiety as a contestant decided that the price of a five-piece bedroom suite trumped a fully loaded, top-of-the-line motorcycle. Their outbursts of excitement became my own as contestants accurately calculated the price for a round-trip vacation to Greece. I also felt the deflation in their emotions as they relied on audience participation for pricing products, only to hear that the figure they selected was too high. The cheering fans pushed them to accept a particular price point. When the final assessment was made, however, the game show host woefully announced that the contestant had been ill-advised, and the price was ultimately too high.

Women, more than any group of people on the planet, have a keen understanding of the agony and ease of paying out-of-bounds prices. We have wanted to kick ourselves for purchasing a pair of pumps on Wednesday, only to realize that the same shoe is being sold at another local store for 20 percent less on Thursday. Our wrath melts like butter after going home and pairing our shoe with the special outfit. Hair and beauty products are no exception to this rule. We have also been known to easily toss discipline aside for the regularly priced hair and beauty products that promise to go on sale in just a few hours. We may reason that tomorrow's pleasures are still sweet today.

While women may be generally dubbed as shoppers and spenders, statistics reveal an interesting trend. The average Black woman spends three times as much on beauty products compared with other American women, according to the Sheconomy® blog.[1] Many Black women are spending at the rates we do because of our unique hair texture and a legitimate desire to represent ourselves well. I and others, though, have fallen into another camp of spenders. At times we've poured our souls and strewn our worth along checkout counters. Sometimes we buy something we can't afford or don't need to gain what has been freely given. Who knows how much I personally have spent on my hair since my twenties? No matter the year-to-date total, I can assure you I spent far more on a quest for peace about myself. The debt I racked up didn't just show itself in my credit score or bank account balance. The deficit was revealed in the way I cared for myself.

Unless I was bathing or washing my hair, water became my arch enemy. As an adult, I strategically positioned myself at the shallow end of the kiddie swimming pool and dared toddlers to splash me. The goal was to keep my toes completely covered and my hair completely dry. Yes, I went to the pool, but I couldn't chance having a spray of water reach my straightened hair, which had been vacuum-packed in an airtight, rubber swim cap. Outside of being water baptized by immersion in church at fifteen, I honestly can't remember going underneath water in my early years. Prank-dunking and water parks were no-no's and grounds for immediate friendship termination. I had a simple, unspoken rule: I shall not get my hair wet.

With this edict as a backdrop, you can only imagine the insanity that occurred when the weather forecast called for a previously unexpected rainy day. The drama was made-for-TV—and ridiculous! Every raindrop that hit my hair represented a dollar that I would have to spend on straightening. Even the threat of precipitation meant money out of my wallet. Instinctively, I knew that the smell of rain meant limited trips outdoors. If I was caught without an umbrella, I'd grab anything to shield my coif from the elements—plastic grocery bags, newspapers, or even my coat. My body could get wet, but not my hair!

Staying rain-free was particularly challenging when walking with my husband, Kyle. The ultimate gentleman, he knew the drill, and would make his best effort to position the umbrella over my precious straight hair. While grateful for his chivalry, I was also a bundle of nerves, and I'd usually anxiously bark out orders like, "Can you move it here?" Then the rain would come from a different direction, and I'd shriek, "No! Now my sides are wet. I can feel my hair rising!" You'd have thought this was acid rain instead of just water. Truth be told, there was no umbrella large enough to shield me from the uneasiness of having straight hair revert to its natural state.

It's a good thing I never had dreams of being a swim champ. Nevertheless, I had other battles to wage because of my hair and the elements. This battle was not on sea but on land; specifically, at the gym. I was never one for strenuous physical activity, and, during my twenties, instead of pumping iron or doing an aerobics class while I was there, my forty-five minutes in the office gym were spent solely at the juice bar. Sips of my favorite, noncarbonated, healthy beverages were the slow road to health, but fast enough for me. If I did go to one of the pieces of workout equipment, it was to read and catch up on current events. Now, mind you, I was still spending money for perms every four to six weeks. This being the case, at that time, I would never let a workout interfere with my blowout. During my reluctant trips to the gym in my thirties, I exerted the least amount of energy possible. Weights above two and a half pounds were not on the agenda. Sweat-inducing aerobics had to take a backseat. After all, I had spent "all of this money" on my hair and was not going to sweat it out. This nonathletic trend showed up in unwanted pounds and followed me well into adulthood. Not being able to fit into my clothes was the least of my health concerns. I was an asthmatic, and exercising would have increased my lung capacity. I also had a family history of hypertension and diabetes, which certainly would have been helped by exercise, but that never registered on my radar. After all, I was too busy "pampering" myself. The problem, though, is that the self-care was only skin deep.

My former relationship to my 'fro and fitness is not uncommon, according to former Surgeon General of the United States, Dr. Regina Benjamin. She shared similar findings during a National Public Radio interview.[2] "There are studies that show that when we ask women—and particularly African-American women—'Why don't you exercise?' And they would say, 'Well, I just spent a lot of money on my hair, I don't want to sweat.'"

It came as no surprise to Dr. Benjamin that Black women are "emotionally invested" in their hair. She expressed, however, the need to make sure that Black women's investment is not just related to their hair, but also to their overall health. "Hair has always been important to women in general. African-American women, in particular—we spend a lot of money on our hair. We spend a lot of time on our hair. It's important that we look good, that we feel good about ourselves. And our hair is an important part of that," she said. An elevated understanding of the tie between health and beauty is still needed for Black women to reach a point of peace. As Dr. Benjamin noted, our personal state is not just relegated to one area of our lives. "Health is no longer in a doctor's office and the hospitals alone. Health is where we live, where we learn, where we work, where we play, where we pray. Health is in everything we do." It is the choice to maintain health in our finances and fitness that underscores the true degree of peace we have with our hair and beauty.

As I'm on the cusp of celebrating eight years as a *naturalista*, my approach to finances and hair is so very different than it used to be. I'm at the point where I want to preserve my natural curl and only purchase the products that will work for me. My cabinets are not cluttered with unnecessary beauty aids that promise to make me look like someone other than myself. I am still not a swimmer, but I have been known to go underwater—without a swim cap—for family trips to beach. My occasional gym day has turned into a three-day-a-week regimen that I absolutely love. I get joy from working out and getting sweaty. The level of sweat just determines how cute and curly I'll be for the rest of the day. My payoffs have been well-managed weight, normal cholesterol levels, and stronger lung capacity.

Years later, I can honestly say that I've achieved a healthy level of peace about my hair and beauty. I realize that society has an opinion about my particular look that is different than my own opinion. I am not fooled. Both exist. Both are polarized. But I choose to lean into the truth that I'm beautifully brown just the way I am! My definition doesn't come from the outside but from within. The opinions of people begin to fade into oblivion. We are quite comfortable to dismiss the chorus of well-wishers and opt for a solo performance on life's stage. At this self-defining moment, we know that our notes may not be perfect in pitch. Our desire, though, is to strike a chord with who we truly are. The notes in this melody will reverberate in our souls and impact the next generation's score.

When our worth is drawn from a deeper spot, we understand and remind others that hair is great, but it does not make us who we are. We are wonderful whether we have hair or not.

One morning, I woke up and all of the hair on one side of my head was lying on the pillow. I sat there for about one hour, crying and holding my hair in my hand. I didn't think it was going to take my hair. I went to the bathroom, got a razor, and shaved my head. It was the hardest thing to do. At that point, I felt like I had lost everything that identified me as a woman. I shaved my head, put the scarf back on, went back to bed, and stayed there for two days. I didn't know how to handle it.

This is Elaine's story. The stage IV breast cancer survivor bravely recalled the defining moment when she lost her hair to cancer. At this point, everything that defined her femininity swirled down the drain with chemo-ridden strands of hair. Many years later, however, she has recovered all. Elaine's body is cancer-free. Her strength and vitality have returned. This is what Elaine recalled:

I woke up one day and realized the Lord was saying "There is another person in here, and she wants to be free." So one day I said enough is enough, and the main thing is I want to be free. I can't hide behind the track or my hair growing out anymore.

Aware that her hair does not define her worth, she is at peace and proudly sports a sassy bald head.

For some Black women, losing moves us toward a point of gaining courage to accept the treasure within ourselves. There are times when the tranquility comes in celebrating what our losses have left behind. Elaine was left with the truth that her tresses merely adorned her value. She came to terms with who she really is after losing a breast to cancer. My hair peace was revealed through a pattern of dwindling finances and health. Resembling a long-division math problem, the subtractions of these poor choices left me with a remainder of truth. I now know, with certainty, that the best of me was never on my head but rather in my heart.

The long-awaited finish line of peace is not for those who sprint but those who are willing to go the distance during adverse emotional weather and uneven psychological terrain. The trek to loving our natural hair and beauty is akin to a well-paced race. The winners are those who participate and refuse to sit on the sidelines and only lead the cheer for another's victory. The crowning laurel of accomplishment belongs to those who will put their best foot forward.

I wish I could say that I was graced with a victory bouquet after every race I've run. I've conquered and run a steady race to become the best version of myself. My reward: a greater appreciation of who I truly am.

However, my attempts at physical races have left a lot to be desired. My sister and mother still chuckle about my home run that never happened when I was seven years old. While playing a game of baseball during a family vacation, I ran with all of my might around the bases. *I'm moving as fast as I can. I know I can hit the base before the ball does. Yippee! Everybody's screaming . . . they know I can win!* I was right about one thing: my family and friends were screaming. However, their message was not what I thought. They were actually yelling, "Michele, you're running in the wrong direction! Turn around and go the other way!"

With this sterling moment in my sports history, let's fast forward to the summer of 2014. This summer run was yet another reminder that I didn't possess the skills needed to run a physical race. On this particular race day, my fame was fleeting. Everyone eyed me as the camera crew trailed me and the other runners. Beads of sweat recklessly poured down my flushed face. Attempts to keep my kinky curls from tumbling into my eyes barely worked. I tried to compose myself but knew that at some point, I would be asked to speak. The TV camera teetered on the field producer's shoulder. The CNN field producer quickly adjusted the lens so he could capture my entire face. No one else could answer his question but me. No one else did what

I had done. The moment of truth finally arrived. After checking the mic's sound levels, his voice pierced the silence. He put the mic to my mouth. He asked the question that was on everyone's mind.

"Did you finish last?"

Every ounce of my body tried to look dignified. I failed, and laughter took over. My squeaky "Yes" was sandwiched between hearty chuckles and plain ole' embarrassment!

What in the world was I thinking? I had already established that athleticism was not my strong suit. Against my better judgment, though, I decided to make a guest appearance at a local running group event for a one-time trek throughout Washington, D.C.'s renowned Capitol Hill. Everything in my body screamed that I was not marathon-ready, but I gave my word, and there I was. The thick, humid summer air was an indicator that I would have to be well-hydrated if I was going to finish in grand style. *Wow. I guess I should be stretching too? Hmmm. But I did walk from my car to the meeting point. I know that counts for something. I'll just stretch as I run!* Honestly, I would have been just as happy to escape with a lame trot among the cherry blossoms or stop at one of the many food trucks for some chips, soda, or ice cream. *Who wants to spend a Saturday running? Ugh! I said I would, so I will.* My crabbing and complaining fell on deaf ears, because these words never left my mouth. My shrugged shoulders and droopy bottom lip told the story to anyone who was paying attention. Considering the fact that I was a group newbie, I don't think anyone even noticed. The more I blended in, the better. No one would point me out. I could finish this run and start enjoying my Saturday.

I guess we'll be starting soon, I thought, while turning to check out my surroundings. The sweeping view of women doing pre-run exercises was a tad bit intimidating. Clusters of vibrantly colored workout gear and mounting energy caught the attention of errand runners and dog walkers who were out for a leisurely weekend stroll. Before I could snatch another longing look at the fleet of food trucks, the shrill whistle signaled the start of the race. *This is a piece of cake*, I thought as I confidently travelled along the curbs and turns on the Hill. Running with seasoned and first-time runners gave me a boost. I paced myself at the traffic lights, just like they did. I bobbed and weaved among crowds of tourists, just like they did.

This is great. I'm not too bad after all. Whew. The finish line has to be coming up soon. I quickly hit the brakes on the personal fanfare after noticing something in my peripheral vision. *No, that's just a coincidence. Wait a minute. Didn't I just see her? Didn't I just see them?* My voice petered out in bewilderment, but my eyesight was shockingly clear. The reason why I saw the same women over and over again was finally obvious. All of them had passed me on the other side of the course! Seeing them the second time around meant they were headed for the finish line. That explained why there was so much "free room" around me. The crowd didn't thin out because the course was hard. The crowd thinned out because their course was over.

The notoriety of coming in last fizzled shortly after the throngs of "show-off" runners gave me my due applause. Since I couldn't crawl under a rock, I decided to hang around the CNN field producer for a bit. After all, why should I waste a networking opportunity just because I was the official rear guard? We had a nice conversation and exchanged contact information. Even though the footage never left the edit bay, I still reaped the rich benefits of being the "caboose" during my memorable race. Since that day, I've kept my word to keep in contact with the field producer for the purposes of networking. Whenever I send an e-mail, I have the distinct honor of being able to start my correspondences with this phrase: "To refresh your memory, I am the young lady who came in last during the race you covered."

This phrase always brings a warm smile to my lips as I remember a powerful lesson. *The fact that I finished last obviously meant that I started.*

Combing through personal issues is tough for some Black women. No amount of makeup or post-graduate degrees prepared me for the deep-seated issues fueling my mane attraction. I admit that journaling about past root issues and fear triggers made me want to take a rest stop along the way. Sometimes it was difficult to come up for air and see that others were farther along in the journey. I now have a greater respect for the process and the prospect of a timetable that doesn't always stack up to others' expectations. I know that my gradual fall into my complete embrace is coming in phases. Will I be known as the one who finished last? I'm not sure. It's really more important to be known as the one who was brave enough to start.

ELAINE JAMISON'S
Hair Story

ELAINE JAMISON *is Director of the Life After Cancer Ministry at Faith United Ministries, District Heights, Maryland.*

This is not my first time being bald. I first went bald back in 1971, before it really even got very popular. It happened when my children's father was supposed to be giving me a shape-up. He messed up so badly that I was forced to go bald. In the beginning, my confidence was shot. I felt embarrassed and ashamed. I remember I stayed home from work for about one week. I didn't know how my job was going to accept it. As time went on, I knew I had to make a living, so I had to adjust.

After becoming a breast cancer survivor, I started to change. Now my hair was already thin, but after the treatment, I had bald spots on my head. I knew my hair would never grow back there. Only a little section of fuzz remained. I would look at other women's natural hair and start to feel jealous because I just wanted to have my old hair back.

When I did go to my hairstylist, I remember wishing that he had a private room; when he took the tracks out of my hair, everybody could see the bald spots from the chemo. I was so ashamed. I would look in the mirror and wish I could just take off all of my hair. After four years of having tracks in my head, I also started to get concerned about the hair glue going directly on my head; I had no hair to keep the glue away from my skin.

I remember just waking up one day and saying, "Enough is enough. I don't want it anymore. I don't want to hide behind the shame of my hair not growing out full anymore. I don't want to deal with thoughts of being less than a woman." At that point in my life, my hair didn't matter. The only thing that mattered was being free.

Now on Saturdays, I get up in the morning and use my own clippers and shave my head. I put Sea Breeze on for about ten minutes, shampoo my head, shine it up, and put on my makeup. I feel wonderful. I feel so good. I feel so free.

I think society pushes Black women to compete with one another. The competition even goes back to our skin color, the way that we speak, and our hair. Just because society has brought it about doesn't mean that we have to play into it. If a sister has hair that is down to her butt—natural or curly—it doesn't have anything to do with the woman I am. I can still celebrate her!

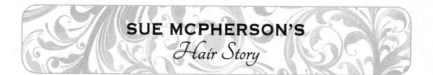

SUE MCPHERSON'S
Hair Story

SUE MCPHERSON *is an indigenous Australian author and visual art-ist living in Eumundi, Queensland. Sue is the 2013 shortlist recipient of the Prime Minister's Literary Award for her YA novel,* Grace Beside Me *(Magabala Books).*

My mum is Aboriginal (Koorie) and Irish; my father was from the Torres Strait Islands off the coast of Queensland. I got my wild hair from my father. As a child, I became a state ward and was fostered and even-tually adopted into a White family. I was given the strong Scottish name of McPherson. My mum, dad, and an Aboriginal sister from a different family lived on the property and went to school in a small country town in New South Wales (NSW). Apart from my sister and me, there were two other Koorie families within the school. The majority of the children in the school we attended were White and of European descent. Unfortunately, I was the only one who had frizzy hair.

When I was a school-aged girl, *Charlie's Angels* was big on TV, and Far-rah Fawcett was the bomb. My poor mum and I spent hours trying to iron my hair. We even tried straightening it and flicking it at the sides; that style just wasn't meant to be. My hair definitely had a will of its own! There was not going to be a Black Farrah Fawcett in country NSW, Australia. Madonna came on the scene later, but I still got no help trying to match her hairstyle. Now, when Miss Whitney Houston hit the charts, I still had no help, because Whitney wore wigs and extensions. Wigs and extensions were totally out of the question for several reasons. First, we didn't have them. Second, they were too expensive. Third, we would have to get them sent in from the

United States. Finally, I'd be laughed at something bad, because everyone would know I was wearing fake hair.

I received plenty of name-calling over the school years, especially up to the age of sixteen. Not only did I have mad hair, but I was also darker than most. So I had no boyfriends through school; I was just too different. I still remember the instigators. I'll never forget the insults, but I'm okay. I made it through, and to this day have many wonderful White school friends who continue to be caring, loyal, and supportive.

I didn't feel comfortable with my hair until about sixteen years ago, when I was diagnosed with breast cancer. When Jesus says, "Hello, I may be seeing you sooner than later," it's a huge wake-up call. Even though the whole cancer show is so destructive—emotionally and physically painful—I believe it was my time. I lost all of my hair—chemo saw to that. When treatment was completed and my frizz grew back, I knew things had changed. My poor old body chugged along 24/7 trying to fight the disease and the horrors of chemo and radiation. With all that my body was fighting against, here I was wishing that my hair was straight. What an immature and ungrateful thing to say. So from then on, I decided to love all of me and not care what anyone thinks or says about me.

For the last three years, I've been blessed with a grey patch at the front of my head. Other grey hairs have joined the party, and they're here to stay. I don't want to dye it. It's natural, and it is what it is. I love things outside the square, so I reckon a funky haircut and deadly outfits will help keep my looks updated. By the way, my handsome hubby is White and of English descent. Given the fact that no White boy wanted to go out with me when I was younger, hanging with hubby makes me proud. He has never questioned my looks. He just loves me for me, with my frizzy grey hair and all.

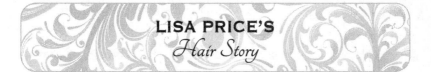

LISA PRICE'S
Hair Story

LISA PRICE *is the founder and president of the multi-million dollar line of Carol's Daughter hair and beauty products. In 2014, Carol's Daughter was acquired by L'Oréal; Lisa remains very involved with the company she started.*

Since I have to represent the Carol's Daughter brand, I actually take care of my hair differently. Before—when I was someone who went to work every day—I would braid my hair a lot or wear twists. I never thought anything of it. My hair grows notoriously slowly, and I would wear these styles to give my hair a rest. Now that I sell Hair Milk on the Home Shopping Network, I need my curls. I make choices with my hair based on the fact that I'm a public person. I don't want someone to look at me and think, "She's selling a product, and she doesn't wear her hair curly?" It's kind of hard to be that chameleon with my hair because of what I'm selling. I kind of have to *be* my brand all of the time.

Feelings about my hair started at home. I didn't grow up feeling like there was something wrong with the hair on my head. What I think my family did for me was give me a different view of my own hair and a relaxer. Some of us used a relaxer for easier styling and manageability. We didn't feel the need to alter what we looked like to conform to a particular image. It was about how much quicker we could get ready in the morning. We just considered how much time it was going to take to do our hair.

When I was growing-up—because my hair texture is a softer grade—I often heard people refer to my hair as "good hair." It took me many years to find out what that meant. It never impacted my self-esteem. We didn't talk about those things at home. Everybody's hair was their hair. When I heard that phrase in other places, it was weird. I never really embraced it and thought he or she was prettier because their hair was one way or another.

With my daughter, Becca, I want to instill a sense of her natural beauty. I chose to put her hair in locs. I did that primarily because I travel a lot, and I wanted a style that was easier for Dad to maintain when I wasn't there. It's been fun for her because now she has ponytails. Becca said to me one day, "I want my hair to be on my shoulders."

I said, "Your hair will get there one day."

I've noticed that since Becca has started wearing locs, she's already embracing a certain style and texture. She will learn to know that she's beautiful.

I encourage women to be themselves. The woman who has embraced the natural texture of her hair is typically someone who feels free. You have some people who are curious about what their hair will do if they don't relax it. I tend to focus on people making choices that work for them. I never want someone to feel like I'm saying, "You need to stop relaxing your hair. That's terrible for you!" Maybe relaxing your hair is what you need. Maybe you're a person who needs things to be easier for you to manage, and this is something you've done forever. When you look in the mirror, that is the person you are comfortable seeing, and you don't want to be uncomfortable. This is fine. Don't do something because you feel like you are less than someone else. Don't touch up your roots because you feel like there is something wrong with the kink showing through. Do it because it works for you, and you're comfortable with it. In whatever way you care for your hair, do it in a smart, responsible way.

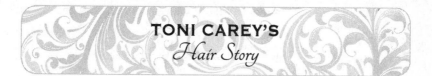

TONI CAREY *is the cofounder of Black Girls RUN! (BGR!), a national running group with more than 52,000 members nationwide. BGR! is the 2014 Oprah's Life You Want Tour Standing O-Vation recipient.*

Statistically speaking, 80 percent of African-American women are overweight or obese. We typically don't put our health before other things. We're taking care of the husband, family, kids, our career. Exercise doesn't rank on our list of priorities. We simply think we don't have enough time to fit in being healthy and everything that a healthy lifestyle entails. Also, exercise is something that is not culturally ingrained in our community. If you were to look at it from a historical perspective, we don't have those conversations about health. I truly believe the lack of discussion about health is the reason certain chronic diseases—like diabetes and high blood pressure—are so prevalent in our communities. We also don't talk about family health history. Typically, we also don't have the education to support making healthy lifestyle choices.

My mom is a hairstylist, so I got my first perm when I was four years old. Hair has always been something that's taken the limelight in my life because I was around it so much. When I started running in 2008, I just found that I couldn't pay someone $100 to have a perm and sweat it out. I was actually inspired by my business partner, who had gone natural the previous year. I thought, *I'm married. My wedding photos look great. Let me just do this now and see what happens.* So I actually cut off all of my hair.

When it comes to working out and being concerned about your hair, I think you have to have some sort of epiphany. You have to see that health is more important than your hair. It takes some people longer to get to that point than others. This realization doesn't always mean going natural. It doesn't mean one thing or the other. It really means that you finally have found a way to do both. It means being able to strike that balance and find something that works for you. The balance may be a weave or perm. It could be going natural, but you can't just say, "I don't want to mess up my hair," throw up your hands, and walk away. That line of thinking—to me—is a sorry excuse.

The process of accepting my hair has been a real journey. It has been emotional. I tell people all the time that it took some time to actually look in the mirror and say, "I like my hair." I'm finally starting to accept it, and this path is part of personal growth. I think you have to go through this process to really know your value and beauty. We just want to put ourselves in a box (i.e., I'm natural, I'm not natural). It's so much more than that. We, as Black women, don't have to let these things define us. That has been the biggest blessing for me.

Combing Through Chapter 5, Hair Peace

Explain your definition of "peace." Are you at peace with all of yourself or parts of yourself? How did you reach this level? How can you experience a greater level?

_____

_____

What role—if any—do exercise and healthy eating play in your overall beauty regimen?

_____

_____

Is your relationship with finances, food, and fitness healthy or unhealthy? Explain why.

_____

_____

What is the "best part of you" that you can offer to the next generation?

_____

_____

Jot down some kind words—or _hairlooms_—about your hair.

_____

_____

Challenge yourself to compliment someone else using your own kind hair words! What are some of the things you might say?

_____

_____

Diagram Your "Mane" Issue

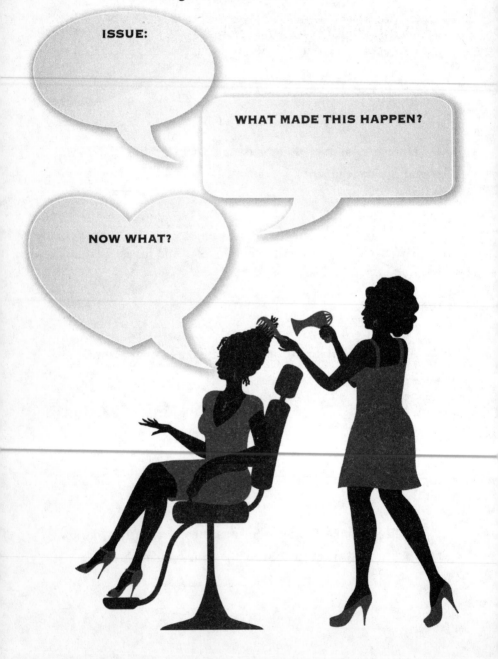

New Growth: Chart Your Solution

Now What?	What's the Effect?	What's Your Solution?

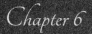

Chapter 6

PONY TALES

L ong before I saw Manhattan's formidable Twin Towers or the Empire State Building, as a little girl I got a personal glimpse of an equally notable high-rise in my South Bronx neighborhood. Those iconic Manhattan buildings, which attracted visitors from around the globe, were no match for what I beheld every summer in my neighborhood. My skyscraper boldly extended beyond the crown of my fuzzy five-year-old head and blocked the scorching fireball of the summer sun. With every ounce of bravery, I would stand on my tippy-toes and briefly peer above the highest point of this tower before quickly losing my balance. My childish determination made me think that I could scale its height. *I'm gonna do it this time! If I pull my head back just a little bit more, I know I can see over the top,* I would always tell myself. Wishful thinking never made my tiny legs stretch enough to lift my gaze beyond the apex of each soaring story.

Now, these stories could have never been reached with the mere push of an elevator button or a determined jaunt to the nearest escalator. Access, though, was always granted to anyone with a mile-high imagination and unbridled creativity. Bound yet liberating, the stories of which I speak were formed by my towering stack of library books!

My mother had an unquenchable thirst for knowledge that she transferred over to me and my sister Sheila during multiple trips to the Melrose Branch of the New York Public Library on Morris Avenue and 162nd Street in Bronx, New York. As soon as my little four-year-old fingers could steady a pen in my left hand, I printed my best oversized letters and became a proud, card-carrying member of the library. On that momentous day, I raised my chubby right hand and pledged to handle each treasure trove with great care and the utmost respect. I secretly issued a cease-and-desist order against the urge to indiscriminately scribble on the books (as I had done on some tables, living room furniture, and bedroom furniture at home).

Always glad to see the library checkout counter, I was equally irritated by yet another library rule. "Now, Michele, you can only take out four books at a time," the librarian and my mother always reminded.

Hmmph! *I don't know why I can't get more. I know I can read more, so why can't I take more?* I'd say to myself.

Rules or not, I was prepared to push the envelope by using my best whine-and-beg routine. In a few instances, a pouty lip and a tilted head did the trick. The next thing I knew, the librarian gave me the thumbs-up, and I gladly charged out of the library with a stack of seven books in tow. As we walked along the uneven city streets, I sure was glad that Mother always brought bags to tote our books across the long city blocks and up the windy staircase to our five-story walk-up apartment. Once inside my bedroom, I hurriedly emptied the bag of books and let them topple onto the bottom bunk bed that was lined with my omnipresent doll collection.

"I know I said I'd play with you, but you just gotta wait," I'd say to my fictitious friends. "Don't cry. I'll get back to you later, but not now!" Baby Alive, Drowsy, and Baby-That-A-Way had no choice but to make room for my new summertime friends. Reading excited me in a way that playing with dolls did not. My head swirled with excitement from trying to pronounce silly Dr. Seuss rhymes. My eyes grew wide with wonder as I lifted each page of Maurice Sendak's *Where the Wild Things Are* and climbed inside each brightly painted character and phrase. A romp inside of Crockett Johnson's *Harold and the Purple Crayon* drew me away from any ounce of boredom and stretched my mind beyond the point of recognition.

Even though I could read by the time I reached kindergarten, there was still something special about having Mother read to me. Her firm yet kind voice made otherwise flat stories burst into colorful dimensions that left me with lasting impressions. Certainly every child has a go-to book during his or her story time. Some children want to hear about ballerinas, trains, or silly characters from now until eternity. While precious in the moment, the time does come when guardians and parents usually get *sick* of reading "that" go-to book. Well, I was no different, because I did have a go-to-book. For the life of me, I can't understand why I felt the need for Mother to hit the repeat button when reading this little book about pancakes.

To this day, we can't remember the name of that book or its author. I do remember, however, that my appetite was profoundly affected after each and every reading. I eventually begged my mother to make me a plate of pancakes after hearing yet another encore performance. My plan worked just as I had hoped. While my mother thought that an ice-cold Popsicle was a better pick for scorching summer days, she nevertheless fired up the griddle and made me a child-sized stack of piping hot, golden brown pancakes, which I gladly gobbled down. Pancakes were the perfect treat for me and made me forget about how steamy it was outdoors and in our apartment without air conditioning. The gooey maple syrup just hit the spot. At five years old, I eventually lived what had been read. I eventually saw what had been said.

This sweet pancake story speaks to the power of a tale that is repeated. My muscle memory jerked and grabbed at the images until they leapt from the pages. I craved what was repeatedly read. The allure of this tale made me believe I should have what I heard, even if someone else had to help me get it. The name of the storyteller or the book's title is not always important. If you are within earshot, a tale's haunting influence can cause your mind to paint pictures that gradually color your palate. The power of repetition affects what lines the mind rehearses and the body performs. I heard the pancake story for a just a few nights and—after four decades—the memory of what happened is as fresh as the moment it occurred.

What transpires, though, when you listen to a tale for years? What will you stomach after feasting on the same story from dusk 'til dawn? Will your movement reflect the word-sketched images? Will the story's grip be sustained if the narrative says you possess superhuman power and indescribable beauty? Will you still live out the tale if it paints you and your descendants as vile creatures who are worth less than horses or ponies?

Like a pebble on a pond, the uncultured and coarse 1712 *Willie Lynch Letter: The Making of a Slave*[1] has caused ripples for centuries. While troubling to read, his story pierced the soul of a nation and caused a systematic departure from the freedoms upon which it was founded. The British slave owner in the West Indies, Willie Lynch, told a tale that has helped steer our nation toward making distasteful actions palatable, one reading at a time. Willie Lynch is said to have spoken these hateful words on the James River bank in the colony of Virginia in 1712. History suggests that colonists asked this British slave owner in the West Indies to share his dehumanizing slave training techniques while there. His namesake: the treacherous act of lynching.

It is human nature to take inspiration from the world around us. Inventions and principled beliefs are often shaped by what preexisted them. The power of draft horses gave birth to the term that defines a unit of power equaling 550 foot-pounds per second: *horse power*. The unsuspecting champion who takes the crowd by storm is often referred to as the *dark horse*. If your claim to fame is a single but stunning skill or trait, you could be seen as a *one-trick pony*. The horse and pony have obviously provided the pool from which people through the centuries have drawn next-level innovation and imagery. In the midst of these analogies, I'm still baffled by the ease with which Lynch and others could look at the human connection with the horse and pony. Unlike the other parallels, his ingenuity did not foster a deeper admiration for the correlation between humans and these animals. Alternatively, Lynch's brand of distortion placed the animal and human on an unnatural, unequal footing. Repurposed, the horse became more than the carrier of goods or transportation for colonial aristocracy. The horse also became the prototype for recasting the role of a sector of the human race. The horse and pony's elevation, unfortunately, precipitated the degradation of Black people.

Let us make a slave . . . we will use the same basic principle that we use in breaking a horse, combined with some more sustaining factors. What we do with horses is that we break them from one form of life to another that is we reduce them from their natural state in nature. Psychological and physical instruction of containment must be created for both. I have a foolproof method for controlling your black [sic] slaves. I guarantee every one of you that if installed correctly, it will control the slaves for at least 300 years. Take this simple list of differences and think about them. Pitch the dark skin slaves vs. the light skin slaves, and the light skin slaves vs. the dark skin slaves . . . whether the slaves have fine hair, coarse hair.

The black slaves after receiving this indoctrination shall carry on and will become self refueling and self generating for hundreds of years, maybe thousands. If used intensely for one year, the slaves themselves will remain perpetually distrustful of each other.

I don't know if we really understand that the fabric of our lives is woven by a tale that was spun centuries ago. For most of us, the view we have of our own hair and beauty was set in motion by a story that was told to us once upon a time. Homespun tales of horror and shame have woven their way into our familial tapestry and will undoubtedly create the fibers of our perceptions. Glances, code words, and nonverbal body language about our hair and beauty don't just mysteriously appear. Often, they are markers deliberately placed in the proverbial history book. These tales have surreptitiously climbed the trunks of our family trees, shaded their boughs, and tainted their fruit.

The slaves were no different. As the years toiled on, I imagine it was easier to forget the realities of our royal African ancestry when society—wittingly and unwittingly—deemed us worthless as a race of people. As Black women were forced to forego ornate African head wraps for common head rags, I imagine that our identity as slaves took shape. As prestigious tribal marks were upstaged by shamefully deep lash marks, the tale stealthily transitioned from fable to fact. It was rehearsed amidst blood-curdling cries and night terrors. White masters and mistresses read the story. Little White girls and boys read the story. As we listened, we learned. As we learned, we unlearned. When the days broke and the nights fell, we listened. As boll weevils wrestled with slaves' blistered fingers for rights to a bale of cotton, we listened. While lynched bodies dangled like rotting fruit from a tree, we worked, and we listened. As the dust of centuries settled, we were still at the feet of masters. We had done more than listen. We had become.

You can always discover a story's transcendence by studying the audience's response after the words are spoken. Captive listeners are thrust from shadow to show based on what they do after they've heard. Holiday dress-ups and sleepovers featuring storybook char-acters disclose who has internalized a story's characters. Without a single word slipping beyond closed lips, the apparel and actions reveal who has become one with the storyline. Historical documents and data make the case that Black and White Americans lifted Lynch's tale from the pages and made it personal. White masters spent most of their lives trying to inculcate Black slaves with the well-worn story. Blacks were forced to dance to the syncopated meter of each word. The message between each line was simple yet complex: Black men, women, and children are worth no more than the horse.

Meanwhile, wicked and vile repetition of the words and imagery made it easy for the audience to rehearse the lines. Lina was born into slavery in Georgia in the nineteenth century. At the time of her birth, stories about the value of Blacks were well-traveled along their generational family lines. If you examine how Lina expressed herself, it is undeniably clear that the lens of her self-image was tinted and tainted. Take a moment to just pore over this ninety-year-old woman's words, and you'll know what tales she'd been told:

> *I is Lina. I 'members all 'bout slavery time, 'cause I was right dar. Course I warn't grown up, but I was big enough to holp Great-granny Rose look after all dem other slave chillun whilst deir mammies and daddies was in de field at wuk.*
>
> *Marster loved to come out on Sundays to see us chillun git our heads combed. Honey d'ere sho was hollerin' on dat place when dey start wukin' on us wid dem jim crow combs what was made lak a curry comb 'ceppin' dey warn't quite as wide acrost. When dem jim crow combs got stuck in dat tangled, kinky wool, damn if dem chillum didn't yell, and Marster would laugh and tell Granny Rose to comb it good.*[2]

Undone hair was not all that Miss Lina and others had to address. Snarly hair often covered the tensions between perception and reality that needed to be uprooted. Tangled perceptions would not be unraveled in one setting. Disturbing at best, every role was filled by a cast of characters with well-rehearsed responses and reactions. Tragedy became comedy, and villains emerged blameless. Wearing rags and living in squalor, we feel the reach of this tale. It had clawed its way from the lips of the narrator and eventually affected how Miss Lina and other slaves—like Miss Jane Mickens—viewed their outward appearances:

> *In dem times ef a nigger wanted ter git kinks out'n dey hair, dey combed hit wid de cards. Now dey puts all kinds ov grease on hit, an'*

buy straightenin' combs. Sumpin' dat costs money, dat's all dey is, old fashioned cards'll straighten hair jess as well as all dis high smellin' stuff dey sells now.[3]

Would it be unfair to say that Misses Lina and Jane's expressions and comparisons stemmed from tales that they heard? Perhaps around-the-clock reminders about the essence and image of Black slaves completely shaped what they saw and how they moved, as well as their views of their abilities, talents, and dreams. These *pony tales*, no doubt, even shaped their views of their hair. Today, you and I would likely do more than raise an eyebrow if someone wanted a ringside seat while we detangled our hair. No words can describe the backlash that someone would get at the mere suggestion that we—like Misses Lina and Jane—should comb our hair with a "card," which is an implement that is used to groom the fur or hair of the sheep or horse. Women may share an outfit or even a piece of jewelry with another woman, but we would be hard-pressed to share our hair comb with another woman. Given an ultimatum to share our comb with an animal or use the same comb it used is unthinkable.

Sharp lifestyle changes usually don't happen unless they are provoked. Tragedies or triumphs can provide the perfect detour along life's road. I'm pretty sure that words like *kinks, wool,* and *nigger* didn't just become part of Misses Lina's and Jane's lexicons. It's no secret that our views can easily change when our environment is altered.

I always loved mood rings as a girl. It seemed like everybody was wearing them in the seventies, and I wanted to be cool, too. I was completely mesmerized by the instant color change once I placed the ring on my fingers. The featured color of the moment always boggled my mind. I figured blue would be next, but green would appear. I'd look for green, and then I'd find the colored stone had unsuspectingly turned to a deep purple. I never quite figured out how the ring's stone could instantly trade off shades of teal for emerald green. With the advent of the color-changing nail polish, my curiosity was raised yet again. This time, though, I finally understood what was taking place beneath the surface. The change in temperature was actually causing the color or "mood" to shift. Nail tips that had been painted lavender turned green once they were were dipped in warm water. It was clear that the color-shifting mood ring was only responding to the change in body temperature. The changing environment—the heated water or elevated body heat—was enough to alter the color of the nail tips and the mood ring.

If inanimate objects can change with rising temperatures, we have to understand that the scorch of slavery's heat was enough to singe ties with the vibrant colors of our culture and heritage. For many slaves, their once-hopeful moods about personhood, hair, and beauty never transitioned into dark shades of midnight. The heat continued to intensify, so the original colors never changed.

We know the story all too well
While others died, some lived to tell
Of broken backs and aching hands
Longing for a place to land
In cotton fields . . . strung up trees
Others caught . . . yet none were free
Spinning fabric . . . telling tales
Best and brightest . . . yet for sale
Born as human . . . viewed like mares
Wool was said to be her hair[4]

As Black women, we still have to do the work of maintaining our true vibrancy in the midst of shifts. Along my own hair journey, there have been instances when I have had to resist my inclination to change my mood or feelings about my hair just because my environment changed. As a college freshman in Central Pennsylvania in the early eighties, I found it hard to locate hairstylists who could care for Black women's hair. I knew that at some point, I was going to need a touch-up, and I couldn't always rely on one of my buddies to apply an over-the-counter relaxer kit! I had already witnessed the epic fail when trying to have a friend give me a Jheri curl in the Black Student Union House. She promised me, "If you put this gel on your head when it's wet, I know it's gonna curl!" After goo-gobs of gel were slathered on my head, the only curl I got was in my neck muscles. I made sure to keep my head hung over the sink while I waited for the curls to appear. Friend after friend would stop by, see me leaning over in the sink and say, "I still don't see any curls." I kept hanging in there, waiting for the best, but I ended up with the worst, which was—in my mind—tightly coiled, puffy hair.

That memory replay was enough to make me go into town and find a professional to wash and style my hair. I had just about run out of options when I decided to go to a beauty parlor near the university. I remember boldly going to a hair salon on the main street of my predominantly White college town. I overlooked the fact that almost every patron stopped to look at me as soon as I walked in the door. Never shy for attention, I figured they must have been taken by my beauty. I knew otherwise but secretly decided to humor myself so that I could walk past some tense moments and piercing stares. Being the center of attention didn't make me lose faith in my assigned stylist's ability to handle my hair. I was, however, ready to hit the door when she came to me with a small, fine-tooth comb and prepared to detangle my shoulder-length hair that needed a touch-up and had about two inches of new growth! At that point, I decided to give her the 101: Black Woman's Hair Styling Course. I gently instructed her to find the widest tooth comb in the shop. I remember her submitting comb after comb for my approval. "No, not that one. Do you have any with wider teeth? Thanks, but that's still not going to work. What other combs do you have? I'd appreciate you bringing those out," I coached. Looking at every comb she had, I finally found something that was not going to leave more hair in the comb than on my head. After that process, I mirrored for the stylist how to gently comb and handle my hair in small sections. We made it through the ordeal, and I wasn't bald when it ended. If you are wondering whether or not I let her style my hair again, the answer is no! Based on how this stylist was noticeably puzzled and uneasy about handling my hair, her jittery moves and shaky hands were a dead giveaway that she was *not* used to washing and styling Afro-textured hair.

Reflecting upon my moments in the salon, I realized, in this instance, that there was no blame to shift or place. What we do is usually an extension of what we know. I imagine that in this city's population of approximately 5,000 people—with less than 5 percent of the population being African-American—that stylist didn't have the need or opportunity to know how to style Black hair. While her understanding may have been limited, I couldn't let her response affect the value I assigned to my hair and beauty.

The decision to embrace who we are is the decision to release the tales and stories told to us that were not true. Bent but not broken, Miss Lina's story as a former slave travels through generations and challenges us to question our own story lines. Who or what has caused our life chapters to introduce us as anemic characters with no beauty beyond what has been assigned? Can you or I charge someone as guilty for making us the villain or victim in our own tale of life? More than 150 years after the Thirteenth Amendment to the United States Constitution (which abolished slavery in our country) was legislated, we as Black women owe it to ourselves to think critically about our next chapters. We can still assume a posture of empowerment when reflecting on how the past has impacted our current hair and beauty choices.

Let's be clear. I have to admit that combing through this segment of American history left my emotions raw and my consciousness heightened. I experienced the edge of tearful moments and fiery rage. With all that has taken place in our rich history, I still know that the answer is not to become a victim. We don't become better by using history as a racial whipping post. Cultural and ethnic contempt never answer the questions that have gone unanswered and unasked. Story lines can begin to be rewritten when we search and grasp for fresh truths while simultaneously releasing old lies.

Miss Lina experienced a lot of loss in her lifetime. There is not enough space and time to chronicle all of the atrocities she and other slaves encountered. Fettered by a debilitating system, portions of Miss Lina's narrative reveal that she did more than spin fabric for her master. Against all odds, she was simultaneously spinning new "fabric" that went against the grain of her imposed view of self and beauty:

Granny Rose larnt me to clean and fix myself up nice, and, Honey, I ain't got too old to primp up now. One thing this old Nigger ain't never done is to put hair straightener on her head, 'cause de Blessed Lord sont me here wid kinky hair, and I'se gwine 'way from here wid dat same old

kinky hair. It's white now, but dat ain't no fault of mine. Honey I sho do
trust dat Good Lord.[5]

Just think: after all of those years of living as a slave, Miss Lina
was able to search through lies and find the truth. It matters not how
long she had to comb through; what matters is that she reached the
breaking point. This is the point where legacy is separated from labels.
This is the point where a pull from the hands of time doesn't take us
back to desolation. Our efforts to switch gears stifle helplessness and
cause bold discoveries to be made. Does Miss Lina's discourse reveal
vestiges of her life as a slave? Of course it does. As we comb toward
freedom, will our discourse reflect shards of an enslaved mindset?
Of course it will. Through this slice of consciousness, we are made
privy to the makings of a new storyline; this new text and tone has
the potential to override the old.

New paragraphs don't always appear in the text at once, but
moment by moment, revelations stand as the editor who skillfully
"redlines" and replaces content. In time, that which was once worked
on in darkness is polished and ready for public consumption.

Among the shells of misfired representations about her beauty,
Miss Lina had the wherewithal to know she could and should "fix
myself up nice." She was expected to die by Lynch's story, but life
slipped in as the tired narrative was read by a new storyteller. Granny
Rose's editorial comments shed new light and gave way to a new
version of a tired tale. The new edition did not fall on deaf ears. Miss
Lina picked up the story and, over time, must have taken it as her
own. The reformed words and images must have resonated, because
in Miss Lina's twilight years, this former slave affirmed, "I ain't got
too old to primp up now."

I wonder what we could overcome if we stepped into storylines that are not widely known? What would we believe about ourselves and other Black women if we dared to peer into a broader historical lens? Perhaps we would see that slavery's descendants birthed daughters who defied odds. These women sidestepped and outpaced lethargic movement toward national change:

- Unparalleled creativity was on display in Italy as Mary Edmonia Lewis[6] did the unthinkable. Born twenty-one short years before slavery's abolishment, she is recognized as the first woman of African-American and Native-American descent to be internationally recognized as a sculptor in the world of fine arts.

- A fresh look through history's pages would explain why bread-making became a lot easier in 1884. Just nineteen years after slavery was abolished, Judy W. Reed[7] became the first African-American woman to hold a patent for an improved dough kneader, the Dough Kneader and Roller.

- From slaves to artisans to inventors, Black women reveal that storylines can be rewritten. Our quest for new story lines may even lead us to Sadie Tanner Mossell,[8] who broke ground in the hallowed halls of academia. Miss Mossell marked history in 1921, as the first African-American woman to earn a PhD in the United States.

Like words on a page, the notes in the scores of our life often need to be addressed and revised. The lives of these Black women have passed into eternity. Their memories prompt us to question the next step in the movement of our lives. The question to us still remains: how can we undo that which has been done? A songwriter since the age of four, I spent hours poring over original lyrics and melodies on my well-weathered, high-gloss kiddie piano. As a preteen, I had long graduated from the flat tones of this imitation baby grand and was diligently playing my apartment-sized upright piano.

Playing the piano and singing my melodies was great, but I wanted to produce. At that age, my allowance of a couple of dollars couldn't stretch far enough for studio time in New York City—or any place, for that matter! In those moments of songwriting, my creativity peaked and reached full throttle. "Money or not, I'm going to record," I declared. "Hmmm, what's the best place for recording? Nah. The sound is great in the bathroom, but somebody's gonna come in," I reasoned. My stroke of genius landed me in the one place of the apartment where no one would even think to look for me. You guessed it; I recorded in the bedroom closet!

Somewhere between the polyester pants, my hot pink fuzzy bedroom slippers, and my playclothes, I found just what I needed. I would squeeze between a bundle of hanging clothes, shut the door, and bask in the solitude of my "it" space near the back wall in the closet. Now, my makeshift recording sessions were never complete without my Sony Walkman Player/Recorder and a blank cassette tape. Both were just what I needed to manually lay tracks and breathe texture into my melodies. Albeit stuffy and warm, the soundproof room made singing and concentration easy. Once I sang the soprano part on side A of the cassette, I would flip the cassette to side B. On that side, I would sing and record the alto part on top of the prerecorded soprano part. After a couple of hours, I finished recording the soprano, alto, and tenor parts. The song was finished, but the melody was fading.

Every time I recorded another voice, the original melody grew fainter. The score was less recognizable. With each flip of the cassette tape, the first melody weakened. Once played for my family, the original version was lost in the last. The end result was a new song;

while different, each additional voice added vibrancy and depth that the original composition lacked.

There are times when we need real healing and transformation by parting ways with outdated words and melodies. New scores are always lingering. They are just a page turn away. While turning the page can evoke fear, life among antiquated stories is far worse. Only you can change the pecking order and priority of what is entertaining and what is irritating. Separation is inevitable. Old tales must reach the end so that new lyrics can soar. Old stories must be shelved, while others can be showcased. No tale ends without a separation. New stories require a split.

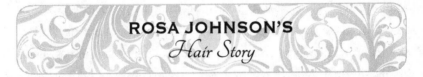

ROSA JOHNSON'S
Hair Story

ROSA JOHNSON *is the niece of the late Dr. Maya Angelou and an experienced archivist. She co-authored* Maya Angelou: A Glorious Celebration *(Doubleday) with Dr. Angelou. Rosa Johnson was also the personal hairstylist and braid artist to Grammy Award–winning singer-songwriter Stevie Wonder.*

I had that hair, what they call good hair. I wore Shirley Temple curls. In the forties and fifties, going to school, I was very dark-skinned and was called "Blackie." I hated it and I would come home and cry in elementary school. My mom would always say, "The blacker the berry, the sweeter the juice." Although I wasn't accepted because of my skin, I had that so-called "good hair." I used it to be accepted into certain groups in school. At first, though, I didn't like my hair and wanted it straightened, but my hair was wavy. I tried to put a perm in my hair once and badly burned my scalp.

When the Black Is Beautiful movement came in, I was in seventh heaven. Not only was I Black, but I was kind of cute! I was in Oakland, California during the height of the Civil Rights Movement. I worked with the Panther Party, and I wanted to be accepted in that group. My hair was a very important part of fitting in. I wanted to look like everyone else, but my hair wouldn't stand up; it was just too straight. I tried everything. I even put mayonnaise on it, but it just wouldn't do it. I remember walking down the street with my daughters, and African-American women would say, "Hey soul sister!" I would say, "Hey," and they would reply, "Oh, not you. The one with the Afro." That comment really crushed me.

It's kind of superficial if you are using how you look to define who you are. It's kind of lightweight. We have to look from where we came to where we are now. We have come a long way, but we need to keep going. Now we feel okay walking around with dreadlocks. Now we are not ashamed because our nose spreads out. We need to keep going and not step back. Focusing on hair is so surface, and we deserve more. We owe it to ourselves, our ancestors, and those who are coming behind. Let that lightweight stuff go. If we don't do it, then what? When you see somebody *go there,* call them on it. It takes a lot of courage because they might talk to you crazy, but call them on it. I think our ancestors—who have gone on and gone through things we could never even imagine—would be ashamed to see how superficial we've become. We have got to rise up. It is time.

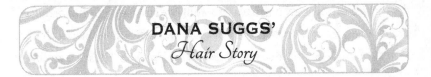

DANA SUGGS'
Hair Story

DANA SUGGS *is the owner of Body and Soul, a cultural boutique located in the center of the Arts District in downtown Winston Salem, North Carolina.*

As a child, I wanted to be accepted and have long ponytails and straight hair. However, I also remember that in the fifth grade, my parents cut my hair so I could wear an Afro. This was a bad time in my life, because I didn't feel attractive. I felt like a boy. When I went back to school, it was confirmed, and I was teased a lot. I was ten years old and I was starting to understand who I was and how I fit into society as a young girl. When I was transitioning from a relaxer as a grown woman, I remember my mother saying to me, "A real woman would cut that all off." When I finally got to the point of actually doing that, it looked like the picture of me when I was in the fifth grade. This time, rather than feeling bad, ashamed, scared, and ugly, I felt so proud and empowered. I really saw a beautiful me that I hadn't seen before. At that point, I saw my real self.

We do judge each other by our hair. It's interesting how that happens. Even now, I will have people come up to me and make comments. They like to ask me hair questions. Now, they love seeing that my hair is natural and that I am confident wearing it this way.

Looking back over my life, I now realize that something happens when you decide to go natural. You may not feel confident because you don't know how people are going to feel about it. You don't know whether they will accept you or embrace you.

The reason why we cannot love and embrace ourselves is based on what we know about our history and culture. I know we are American, but we are African-American. This fact should be reflected in who we are. Everyone else as a race of people is proud of who they are. You see it when you go into their homes. When you go into our homes, though, you don't really see that. We don't know much about our general contributions to the world.

We have to realize that the times have changed. This is a new century, and people are now more accepting of other cultures. Black women should put in the work of knowing ourselves better. We'll then start embracing more things about our culture—our literature, our art, our fashion, our color—and we won't alienate ourselves. We will not only love others but ourselves as well. I think if we totally embrace ourselves confidently, it will also be okay for other people to accept us as well.

I believe that Black women should wear their hair based on what they like. When I was younger and doing the relaxed hair, it was perfect for what I was doing in life and my lifestyle. I didn't think I'd be able to achieve certain things if I had natural hair at that time. Now that I am natural, when I wake up, I know I'm going to have a great day. Now it's really up to me. One thing I don't have to worry about is my hair; it's always fabulous. And to me, that's how I feel. Now, other people may say, "You need to put a perm in." But to me, it's always looking good. This is me, and this is my hair.

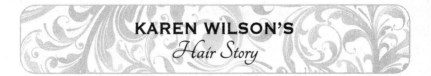

KAREN WILSON'S
Hair Story

KAREN WILSON *is the founder and Chief Styling Specialist of Karen Wilson Natural Beauty—a natural hair care business educating women on the beauty of natural hair. Committed to educating women on loving and styling their own natural hair, Karen developed an educational series called* The Kurl Talk: Learning to Love Your Hair One Strand at a Time. *This series was designed to teach participants about ways to adopt healthy hair by developing healthy lifestyles. Karen's broadcast credits include her features as a regular commentator and natural hair care expert for CBS News WTVR's two-part report on perceptions of natural hair in the African-American and professional community. Karen also teaches workshops at Taliah Waajid's World Natural Hair and Beauty Show in Atlanta, Georgia. She serves on the LB Beauty Education Foundation board as the Public Relations Chairman. She received a dual master's in social work—urban studies degree from Michigan State University, and currently resides and operates her salon in Richmond, Virginia.*

I've always been curious about my hair. I didn't like the styles my mom did; she just kept my hair in plaits. I didn't like that hairstyle, and I didn't think that hairstyle was attractive on me, even at a very young age. I didn't think I was pretty or attractive because of my hairstyle. I didn't link my beauty to my hair texture, because it was always straightened or in plaits. When I was ten years old, my mom said, "Okay, Karen, you can do your own hair." That's when my passion and love for my hair took off. I enjoyed it. I loved the creativity that developed from doing my hair; I could do so many things with it.

When I took care of my hair, it was relaxed, and I gradually started to notice my hair had thinned out over the years. At the age of thirty, I looked back at a picture of me when I was about twenty-five, and my hair was thicker and longer. Since I knew I had not changed my hair regimen, I attributed the hair thinning to the relaxer. I also began to realize that I had no idea what my hair looked like natural. I didn't want to spend my whole life covering up that part of me. I wanted to know what my hair looked like when it came out of my scalp, so I cut it off. Even though I cut it all off at one time, it took me two years to actually do that. I had to change my mindset. I made the mental change first, then the physical.

Before cutting my hair, I never really had any major struggles with my image, appearance, or body. When my hair was short and relaxed, I embraced myself because this style was acceptable. When I cut my hair and wore a Teeny Weeny Afro, or TWA, though, I started to struggle emotionally. This was a challenge for me. As a stylist, I embraced my hair immediately; I picked up the different styling techniques very quickly and easily. On a more personal level, I had to learn to relove my new image.

Since I've been wearing my hair in its natural state, now I know that true beauty radiates from the inside out. Hair is a physical attribute, and regardless of whether it's short or long, or curly or straight, you are still beautiful because God created you, and He does not make any mistakes. My favorite scripture is Psalm 139:14: "I am fearfully and wonderfully made; Marvelous are Your works." Love yourself first, and everything else will follow. It doesn't matter what your hair looks like; God created you, and you are beautiful, gifted, and talented. The emphasis should be placed on who you are and not what you are, in terms of hair.

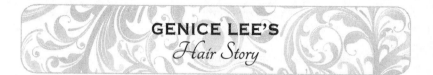

GENICE LEE'S
Hair Story

GENICE LEE, *owner of Harvest Estate and Appraisal Services LLC, lives in the Washington, D.C. metropolitan area, where she works as an appraiser and estate consultant. She has completed appraisals for pieces that have been gifted or loaned to institutions such as the Smithsonian Museum of African-American History and Culture, the Doleman Black Heritage Museum, and the National Canal Museum. Genice has a BA in Japan Regional Studies from the University of Washington and an MA in International Communications from the American University. An accredited member of the American Society of Appraisers, she serves on the public relations subcommittee. Genice is a past president of the Washington, D.C. chapter.*

I can remember that when I went to Japan in 1985 as an exchange student, my hair was truly a fascination and mystery to the Japanese. In Japan, there is a lot of emphasis placed on everyone *being alike*. Of course, being African-American, I stood out, but then to have my hair in braids made me stand out more. I would walk down the street, and people would stop and boldly stare. I remember going to the store to purchase something for lunch, and out of the corner of my eye, I saw this hand reaching out for my hair. I stopped and said in Japanese, "Don't do that!" I had the opportunity to travel to Thailand, and they were also amazed by my hair. A woman from Thailand offered to braid my hair, but I said no.

I remember the anguish I experienced when I was deciding what I should do with my hair when I was there. At that time, there was no one in Japan who could chemically treat my hair. I can recall what I went through trying to get my hair dyed and actually having someone try to translate. I had taken a hair dye kit with me, and one of my teachers tried to translate to a Japanese person how to color my hair. The stylists didn't know what they were doing. By the time I returned from my trip, my hair, which reached past my shoulders at one time, broke off from the humidity and poor styling experiences. I eventually had to get my hair cut very short. When I returned to Japan in 1991 to teach English as a second language, I made a decision that I wasn't going to let anyone do anything with my hair! At that point, I began to wear braids with the extensions. I learned how to braid my hair myself and began to wear it that way.

I can recall that at one time, I did braid my hair and put beads in it, which is very normal for an African-American woman. My choice to wear beads in Japan, though, created such a stir and commotion at the school. The situation reached a point where the teacher who was assigned to take care of me came to me and asked me to take the beads out of my hair.

In hindsight, I find it ironic that in my transition stage, I decided to wear chemically treated curly hair. I did that because I wanted my hair to be curly and didn't realize that my hair is naturally curly. It took me until my late thirties or early forties to have the patience to learn about my hair. I learned to respect and manage my hair to emphasize the curliness of my hair, which I now love. When I was younger, though, I tried to achieve what I already had through chemicals.

I have heard it said that a woman's hair is her crown and glory. I think that we in the African-American community have let people outside define what is beautiful for so long. Embrace the hair that you were naturally given. The hair that you were given is not a mistake. As long as you are okay with your hair, others around you will learn to be okay with your decisions.

Combing Through Chapter 6, Pony Tales

What tales and stories have affected the feelings you have about your hair and beauty? What did you hear? What did you eventually believe?

_____

_____

What role—if any—have you played in your own healthy perceptions about your hair and beauty?

_____

_____

Who do you admire as a role model for healthy hair and self-esteem? Explain your answer.

_____

_____

Fill in this blank: I would love myself more if I changed the way I feel about my _____! Are you willing to make a change? How can you rewrite old storylines about yourself?

_____

_____

Jot down some kind words—or _hairlooms_—about your hair.

_____

_____

Challenge yourself to compliment someone else using your own kind hair words!

_____

_____

Diagram Your "Mane" Issue

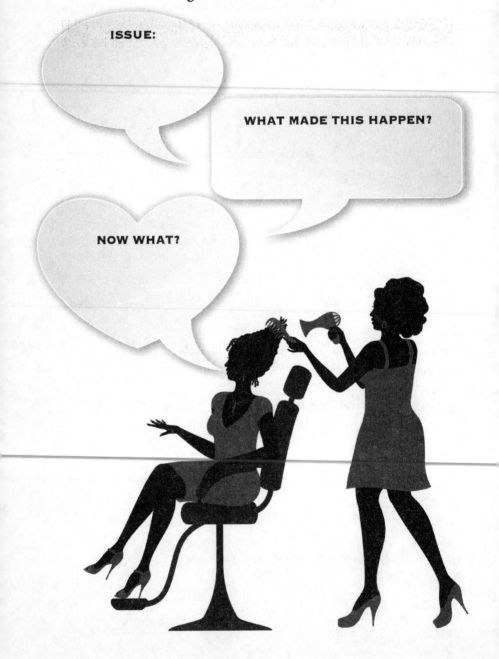

New Growth: Chart Your Solution

Now What?	What's the Effect?	What's Your Solution?

Chapter 7

THE SPLIT ENDS

I heard the legend crumble.

The weight of his fall quickly hijacked the silence of the peaceful, tree-lined campus sidewalk. A few feet ahead of me, the crashing sound was indistinguishable, yet held me captive. My heart raced as I got closer to the sound where, just feet from the scene, the mystery was solved. The deafening commotion was the sound of an elderly man slamming into a metal mailbox.

Anguish and shock were scrawled across his well-weathered face. The steady hand that often penned well-balanced columns now frantically grabbed for anything to make him stable. His desperate attempts to break the fall just weren't working. He buckled at the knees and repeatedly banged against the mailbox post. Words slipped out between shallow gasps for air, but I knew the story.

This veteran journalist was having a heart attack right before my eyes.

Mere moments earlier, I sat mesmerized by his rousing lecture to me and other fledgling reporters. I decided to follow in his footsteps after the class ended. Little did I know that my plan to trail him to get the interview would position me to see this nationally recognized columnist teeter between life and death.

As he clutched the mailbox, it became very clear that I had to make a split-second decision. *What do I do now? I can't believe this is happening. Wait . . . didn't I just see him standing and joking a couple of seconds ago? He looked like everything was okay. This can't be happening,* I thought. *What am I supposed to do? I can't save a life. Where's campus security? Where is everybody? I don't know what to do.* These panicked, rapid-fire questions were coupled with thoughts about what this moment could mean for my career. What up-and-coming reporter would pass an opportunity to tip the media to this story? Already in the nation's capital, American University is strategically placed in close proximity to an NBC affiliate and innumerable media outlets. I was sure that giving this story to the campus paper would quickly leak to local and national press; my career would forever be set.

These images of grandeur and promotion quickly faded. In the midst of my dizzying tailspin of "what ifs," I found myself riveted by an image more powerful than my vision. As we locked eyes, I was drawn to this struggling legend's face. In that instant, I realized that I was not just looking into the eyes of a cherry-picked opportunity. I understood I was looking into the eyes of a son, a husband, and a father. I was looking into the eyes of someone who—beyond the coveted accolades and achievements—was just like you. He was just like me. I was looking into the eyes of a person.

It was this second glance that prodded me to forego any moments of "glory" and hurriedly call 911. As expected, the campus and local emergency medical technicians arrived on the scene. He survived the heart attack, and I learned two lessons. When stripped of our accomplishments, I now know that—at best—we are just people who deserve to be valued and treated kindly. The last lesson still lingers today: the first one on the scene always has a price to pay.

The "firsts" usually shoulder greater weights than their successors. The eldest child may be prematurely pushed to master the ABC's so that parents can have bragging rights. The chore of swimming through a sea of glazed eyes may fall on the first conference speaker. Morning-shift employees usually have to make brimming carafes of coffee before even checking their emails. As seasons take their turn, though, the fruit of early labor appears. Younger siblings glean from a sister's ability to quickly form words. The late-morning speaker reaps warm applause after the keynote breaks the ice. Groggy employees can get a no-effort caffeine fix and begin to work at full capacity.

For many Black women, we have been the first to face issues of hair and beauty. We are those who have been through mounting identity crises that have left us lifeless and limp. Beleaguered by public and private forces, we have sustained blows below the belt about our image and still emerged. Through it all, the eyes of another are locked upon our faces. The youthful stares of our nieces, sisters, and cousins are steadily fixed upon us. Glances and gazes from our community elders and passersby are watching our every move. Imagine how far Black women, teens, and girls could walk if the trail had already been marked by us? No doubt, they could scale greater heights because we had the courage to dig deep. Good or bad, our historical information makes us mission-ready. Our experiences give us a leg up on the next generation.

Like it or not, there is an unshakable responsibility when we are the first to arrive. I never asked to partner with 911 on that day. I still made the choice to do it once I saw the columnist in crisis. Maybe you didn't ask to rescue that friend or coworker during a hair or self-esteem crisis, but she stopped by your desk first. Going out on the proverbial limb may be necessary to reach someone dangling in despair over post-chemo hair loss or alopecia. How can "refusal to resuscitate" be an option when we see hundreds of Black women in our social, professional, and personal circles nearing Code Blue status? How can we witness anemic efforts to cover frail esteems and misshaped perceptions but remain on standby? One hard stare into the face of their realities could be the start of a remedy for this dilemma that we and other Black women face. We are well into the twenty-first century, but the collective health of Black women's self-esteem has not been fully realized in our communities. We see, read about, and have witnessed too many sisters who display a level of self-awareness and self-embrace that is average at best. Beneath our public images, private pains often leak through the seams of our loose-fitting garments of esteem. Only the gaze of intentionality will reveal that there is someone who needs what we have to offer. Our experience may be the missing ingredient for anyone who dares to follow in our footsteps.

As a preteen, I relentlessly begged my mother for a pair of now-vintage Dr. Scholl's wooden exercise sandals. As a recent South Bronx transplant, I desperately wanted to fit in with my lower Manhattan middle school friends. I told myself, *Jessica has a pair, and so does Jamie. I've gotta get my pair next. The field trip to the Bronx Zoo is next week, and I'm already wearing my blue jeans and blue-striped shirt. I know Jason will look at me if I wear those on the trip. I'll look sooooo cute!* My closest friends wore these shoes and, to me, they epitomized haute couture. I was fascinated by the sound that the natural wood sandal made against downtown's cement pavement. Each shoe had the customary, foot-contoured light wooden bottom. The real beauty, though, was being able to select the smooth leather toe strap, which was available in an array of mouthwatering colors. "Now if I get black, that will only go with two outfits. I can't get red because I don't have enough red outfits. Wait a minute. My friends have blue, so we can really look alike. That's the color I really want." After repeatedly hounding my mother, she gave me that for which I had longed. I finally got my pair of Dr. Scholl's sandals.

The only thing that remained was to show them off during my school trip to the Bronx Zoo. I will never forget slipping my foot beneath the thick navy blue strap that was fastened with a shiny brass buckle. I disregarded the facts that the base of the shoe was rock hard and that my feet were flatter than pancakes. As I walked alongside my mother at the zoo, I was swollen with pride—and the swelling quickly traveled to my feet. After walking to see caged apes and talking birds, my once-confident stride turned into a painful hobble. Trailing behind my mother and the rest of my cool classmates, I eventually had to "'fess up." My cringing face and tear-filled eyes were a dead giveaway that my cute shoes weren't as cute as I thought. I never imagined that the shoe I was dying to have was about to kill my feet.

As loving mothers do, mine noticed that my gait moved from a weary trot to a painful drag. Before the tears had an opportunity to crawl down my cheeks, she demonstrated the greatest act of kindness toward me. I never said a word, but she read between the lines of each pain that caused me to wince. She wasn't willing to see me agonize over a poor decision. My mother gave me her shoes and put her feet in mine for the rest of the journey. During her forty-plus years, she had traveled more terrain than I ever had. Her feet had walked roads more hazardous than a city zoo and still had mileage left. Her experience undoubtedly equipped her to handle that which made me limp. Her consistent walk upon harder ground made it possible for my tender, immature feet to handle the next leg of our Bronx Zoo adventure.

Many Gen X, Y, and Z-ers are begging for a brand of beauty that mirrors the hottest looks flooding social media—if even for a split second. The glitter of public acceptance has captivated the young and unaware. Assimilation's shine sends many scrambling for a place to belong. Secret obsessions with particular hairstyles and body images have sent some on the prowl for ways to become anyone other than themselves. As originality is swapped for Instagram filters and Snapchat stories, the next generation is slowly separating from its roots. The bond with their identity and truest essence is dangerously unraveling at the speed of trending topics. Before our very eyes, we are beginning to see metaphorical split ends.

Who doesn't know the perils of split ends? Like a tornado, hairdos caught in the destructive vortex of these divided strands are destroyed. Undone, they cast any hairstyle in the worst light. Now we know that split ends don't just pop up without some assistance. Like accomplices on the crime scene, heated styling tools and harsh chemicals played a hand in the demise of many African-American women's hair. The weapons of the beauty warfare repeatedly zap moisture from our ends. The hair becomes dry. The follicular bond eventually weakens. Unsuspecting kinks and coils fall prey to multiple attempts at identity alteration. Our strands separate over concerted efforts to create an exterior and interior beauty brand that was never intended.

It could be possible that you and I are the current and next generation's hope of mending the bond. Our personal—albeit small—discoveries could just be what's needed to stop the separation raging within many Black women. For instance:

- *Do I love myself, or do I hate myself?*
- *How can I love myself when I hate my hair and looks?*
- *I love my brains, but I hate my body.*
- *I love your look, but I hate my own.*

I can always tell when my strands are stressed, torn, and damaged. When combing through my hair in this state, I will always end up with multiple knots that I just cannot untangle. No amount of conditioner or gentle picking will work. Wide-tooth combs and Denman brushes don't stand a chance when meeting each snarl. Protein treatments, satin bonnets, and roller sets won't do it. There are times when even our best efforts to mend the tears in our souls leave our hair and esteem undone. At times, these tangles have a way of wrapping around each other and leaving us with only one method of correction. When our figurative and literal "strands" reach this point, the dreaded T-R-I-M becomes the order of the day for split ends.

Now, we all know that it seems to take a century for Black women's hair to grow! The last thing we want to do—even with only two inches of new growth—is cut off even an eighth of an inch. It just takes too long to grow back. A good solid trim, though, is the cut that eventually cures. Breakage that stemmed from tightly wound rubber bands can be restored. Edges once ravaged by brown gel residue can have a fighting chance. Healthier sections of over-processed hair can breathe a sigh of relief and look forward to being full again. Personal trimming may also be painful, but with each snip of an unhealthy behavior or jagged mindset, health can emerge. Whether we decide to extract relationships or negativity from our lives, we are setting the stage for new growth.

Newness will surface after the split, but not without some assistance. Everyone does not have the steady hand needed to trim. Best efforts can easily go south and leave you with an uneven bob or asymmetrical chop. Our Aunties, Big Mamas, and cube mates shouldn't have to go it alone when help is available. I firmly believe the skill needed to help other Black women shape healthier lives takes two sets of hands: theirs and yours. Too often and too quickly, we disqualify ourselves as guides and list our every inadequacy. We take a personal inventory and weigh our deficits heavily. We have not always excelled in our quest to love our hair and beauty, but we do have the "secret sauce" needed for someone else's success. You, my friend, have experience!

Do you realize that someone is destined to cross a path that we have already chartered? Whether desired or despised, I know for a fact that my hits and misses have been the great connector for someone who is not quite at my spot on the quest for acceptance. I'm amazed that my decisions to uproot personal issues of hair and beauty catch the attention of complete strangers. My coily hair has wrapped its way into sidebar conversations at social gatherings. My Afro puff has sparked conversational reminders that natural hair can go to work. Stranger-turned-acquaintances now know my coveted hair tips and secrets. From heat damage to roller sets gone wrong, my decision to comb through is helping other Black women to make it through. Your story, too, can easily invite another woman to check her root issues before the core of her self-image completely splits.

Our efforts to help another woman can be met with resistance. The struggle may not come from outside, but from within. Human nature can easily rear its head and snatch the glow of altruism. Tensions generally rise when we catch wind that our assistance means that others get what we've got with less effort. Justified at first glance, we must realize that we may be positioned as the individual to start the change because we're equipped for the job. We also have to consider that we have not always been the one to set the course and help someone along. There were times when we followed the lead of someone whose journey started before ours.

If you unbraid the strands of your life, it won't take long to realize that someone had a hand in pushing you closer to the front. A hand has always guided us along each phase of our lives. The fingers of disciplined mentors course-corrected our blunders and missteps. Teachers or beauticians needled us until we traded toxicity for health. Sista friends, buddies, and strangers applauded our well-done efforts and moved us toward the winner's circle. From C-suite connections to awkward first kisses to bargain basement sales, we have always needed a hand to lead the way. We may be first today. Only moments ago, though, we were the ones who followed.

The walk along our stony road can pave someone else's path. The less experienced will have to comb through issues just like we did. With a little insight and wisdom from us, though, their detangle time can potentially be cut in half! Our decision to witness the damage and assist with repairs is really where the split ends.

I learned, after witnessing the journalist's heart attack, that it's never enough to see. I had to stay. I'm not sure how many moments passed before the emergency responders arrived. Jokes and chatter were suspended in mid air because my time was being redirected.

Moments of going to the study lab and penciled-in appointments were shifted because crisis closure takes time. I always say, "Change doesn't come overnight, but it will come over time."

Speaking of time, I couldn't quite pinpoint the time of day when my vision began to change. Throughout my 2015 Thanksgiving dinner in North Carolina, I was able to clearly see shaved slices of honey-brown glazed turkey. The white swirls of cream cheese frosting whipped around moist chunks of red velvet cake; this masterpiece didn't escape my eye. For some reason, though, my vision wasn't quite the same that Black Friday. Just one day after Thanksgiving, and I noticed traces of brown and dark-red streaks dancing before my right eye. While lying in bed, I repeatedly blinked, but the streaks were still there. *I know what it is. I fell asleep and didn't take out my contacts. Now, Michele, you know better than that. Remember what happened the last time. Get up and take these out. You know you didn't wash all of the eye makeup off. That black mascara and eyeliner will do it every time!* I carefully removed the contacts and makeup, but the streaks were still there.

Wait a minute. Something's not right. My eye looks fine. Kyle even looked in my eye, and we don't see anything. Why do I keep seeing these streaks? Okay, Michele, just be cool. Don't panic. After some rubbing, eye rinses, and more stops by the mirror, I knew something had happened to my eye. It didn't matter that I appeared to be fine in everyone else's eyes. Inside—based on what I was witnessing—something had happened to my eye. Something had shifted. Something had changed. After a frantic phone call to my affiliated eye care group, Kyle and I headed to the ophthalmologist. It didn't take long to fill in the blanks of my mind. The ophthalmologist let me know that my view wasn't altered for an external reason. Makeup residue wasn't obstructing my view. Well-worn contacts didn't create a film over my eye. What I saw was the result of something more serious and far-reaching. A blood vessel in my retina had ruptured; I had sustained a retinal hemorrhage.

What happened when we returned to Maryland was nothing short of a whirlwind. Work schedules abruptly shifted, alternate drivers graciously stepped in, and appointments were cancelled indefinitely. Over the course of several months, my right eye experienced more poking and prodding than a piece of prime rib on the Cooking Channel. After multiple sessions of having my eye dilated, I was the proud owner of a small, private collection of unstylish, flimsy plastic wraparound shades.

As I am putting the finishing touches on this manuscript, it is a sheer miracle that my eye is healed. Undoubtedly, I was the first one to arrive on the scene of a personal crisis. After all, it happened to me. The mending and healing happened, not overnight, but over time. Now, I had no choice but to stick around for the months it took for my eye to mend. Where could I go? I am forever attached to my eye! Because of my attachment, my once-cloudy vision is now clear.

We can always choose to run when we see another Black woman who is battling the same mission problems we have encountered. The beauty, though, is staying around for the mending process and refusing to leave. Staying may mean holding someone's hand through the "big chop." Someone else may listen—for the hundredth time—about how your buddy is going to the gym as soon as she gets time. Being available for another Black woman's healing may mean encouraging someone to make food choices that will improve their hair and well-being. We and other Black women did not separate from ourselves all at once. Decision after commitment after choice, the fraying began.

Like clear fingernail polish on the snag in a pair of panty hose, your experience can keep another sister from "running." Give her a chance, and give it some time.

Thankfully, the retinal hemorrhage I sustained mended without medicine. In some instances, more invasive measures are needed. Likewise, the correction needed for my vision may be different than yours or another Black woman's. We can all heal but the path is usually not the same. While the process needed for us to reclaim 20-20 vision will take on different shapes and forms, every plan should include these steps. Let's remember our H.A.I.R. in the healing process:

Healing Usually Comes in Stages

I have always been a ham for as long as I can remember. I never saw a camera that wasn't automatically looking for my face! The stage was the place when I seemed to come alive. Now, in most instances, I wasn't cast in pop-up performances. I knew well in advance that I was about to mount the stage. What did I do? I rehearsed my lines. I figured out what I would say and how I would react to the crowd and manage my nervous quirks. Gradually—after all of the preparation—I was ready to go public.

Similarly, the hemorrhage was deep-seated and wasn't going to heal in a moment. I had to get used to blinking and seeing bright blood stains. At the next stage, I would blink and notice the bright red stains were deeper brown. The next stage meant blinking and seeing streaks that had turned into only dots or specks. In the final stage, I was able to see clearly. For a lot of Black women, our wounds are deep. We've got to blink a few times and practice saying some new lines about ourselves. After some time passes, we'll blink and actually smile when we see our true beauty. We will refuse to engage in self-criticism. At some point, we will reach the stage where we embrace who we are from the inside out. Our ability to do that is based on the following thought.

Accept What You've Got!

Who would have ever thought you would have multiple textures of hair on your head? Perhaps the hair around the napes of our necks and edges is more tightly curled than the hair at the crowns of our heads. Maybe your friend's hair is straight all over, and she's never had a kinky strand in her life. Whatever we've got, at some point, we have to just move forward. Our hair doesn't need *coarse correction*; we just need to accept what we've been given. We can ogle someone else's accomplishments, strain to get someone else's body type, or wrestle with what has been squarely placed in our laps.

After the retinal hemorrhage, I had to accept the fact that—for a season—I was going to see streaks and spots from the broken blood vessel. I had to get used to having my eyes dilated during countless eye exams. Was it a nuisance? Yes. Did I want to side step the hemorrhage? Yes. But once I accepted the truth and endured the process, I could experience healing.

Let me just ask: how much time do we spend trying to live like someone else? Better yet, how often do we vicariously escape into the people showcased in the most popular reality show or blockbuster movie? How often do we encourage the sisters around us to do the same? A view of someone else's life can be a wonderful way to avoid pitfalls and find solutions to recurring issues. Admiration, though, goes awry when we use it as a means of escape. We'll only

know if we are women who promote avoidance when we consider
the next thought.

Investigate Your Surroundings

Just think for a moment about your last or current love interest. Did
you "go *CSI*" on that person? I know I did when I was first introduced
to Kyle. I had my private eyes planted in strategic locations. I wanted
to see if he was flying solo or if he was already connected to someone
else. Now, before you get ready to judge me, stop one minute! We
all know that we will hit the Internet, credit bureaus, and colleagues
before trusting someone with our e-mail addresses, phone numbers,
and tender emotions. This level of diligence is non-negotiable when
considering who will handle our valuables. When was the last time
that we really investigated how we handle ourselves and respond to
our own image? Are we okay with thinking less of ourselves? Do we
easily allow another Black woman to berate herself in front of us and
not challenge her to see differently?

With my eye, I had to backtrack and explore what transpired
before the blood vessel burst. I've since learned that stress can cause
retinal blood vessels to become damaged and rupture. When I realized why it burst, I had to begin checking myself for stress points. Personal and professional circles were the first places to start. I couldn't
deny it. The evidence had already surfaced, and there was no place
to hide.

Now, let's consider: do you think that stress may have caused some
of us to throw our hands up at being our best and say, "What's the
use?" Maybe the tug and pull of it is causing your associate to sink
into a funk that won't go away. Don't just sit by. Dig around and see

what might be bubbling beneath the surface. Every issue deserves to be addressed. No Black woman's issue is too big. None of your issues are too small. This type of self-care can be summed up in the final phase of our healing process.

Respect Your Progress

If you've never been around a baby who is just taking his or her first steps, it is pretty amazing. They go from crawling, to pulling themselves up, to taking those tentative, clunky moves solo. At best, they may take two steps, fall, and stop—and then the room erupts with thunderous applause. Why? They had the courage to try something new. Admittedly, they didn't get far, but each tiny step taken is a step worth celebrating.

I cannot tell you how psyched I was when I reached the final stages of healing from the retinal hemorrhage. I literally broke down and cried when I blinked and realized the streaks of blood and residue were gone. While my final response was emotional, along the way, I remember becoming my own cheerleader at each juncture. "Okay, this month is better than the last. Thank God I'm only seeing a few streaks!" As progress continued, I said, "What? I get to wait two months before another eye appointment? Awesome!"

When was the last time you celebrated yourself or another Black woman who is taking steps to stop self-deprecation? I hope you didn't throw up your hands and say, "Aw, that's nothing. Everyone exercises. I only did ten minutes on the treadmill. That's no big deal. All I did was drink more water and make sure I tied up my hair at night." These steps may be small, but if we keep making them, over time, we will reach our individual and collective goals.

Any move we make to truly love our natural hair and beauty is worth the effort taken. It's dicey, of course, but the option of inactivity falls flat as we recognize what is ours to gain or lose. Beyond neatly brushed baby hairs and diligently checked roots, a decision to love ourselves through fears and ill-formed attractions can change everything we've known about ourselves and others. Untethered by obstructed views, pressing forward frees us to conquer emotional terrain that was once off-limits.

Each step that we and other Black women take is akin to the way a weaver of fabric uses the loom. When a new tapestry is created, a loom is the tool used to keep new threads in place during the weaving process. Each solid insight provides the balance we need to begin overlapping new strands of truths with tattered strands of lies. The dull colors of outdated words are intertwined with the depth and vibrancy that comes from self-discovery. Barely visible at first, our bold efforts are apparent as we take a few steps back. In time, we will be able to realize that new fabric is beginning to take shape and reform our lives. One glance over our shoulder reveals another Black woman who is also addressing critical issues with a bit more agility and poise. A little more distance will prove that strands of clarity and focus are beginning to emerge. Perhaps these strands were there all along. Perhaps we only see them now because we made the choice to comb.

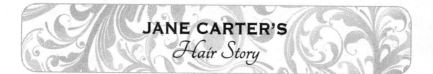

JANE CARTER'S
Hair Story

JANE CARTER *is the founder of Jane Carter Solution and has been a professional hair stylist/colorist and salon owner for over twenty years. Coming from a family of innovators, Jane Carter has become the driving force for a brand that exemplifies a purpose, a cause, and a solution. Jane founded the Jane Carter Solution over a decade ago, after an allergic reaction caused by prolonged exposure to chemicals in traditional hair care products. Life experience contributed to the woman Jane has become: a woman who has spent more than twenty years representing and creating a voice for women. Having suffered family losses due to segregation and racism, her personal life and business model caters to diversity. Being one of the first African-American students admitted into a White elementary school, Jane witnessed community and racial uproars at just six years old. She was genetically wired to fight for the underdog. Frustrated with the lack of chemical-free product choices, Jane decided to formulate her own hair care line using plant-derived ingredients. It is specifically designed for all hair types and textures.*

My family has the whole range of hair textures and complexions. I have always been a rebel when it came to me deciding how I was going to wear my hair. My orientation was developed around a family of women who believed, "Whoever you are is just perfect and who you are." I grew up believing that if you want to shave your head, it's okay. I think that I've always had the freedom to be fully self-expressed. Hopefully, I've done the same thing with my daughters and taught them to have the confidence to simply express themselves just the way they are. I think that you have to do whatever makes you happy. The choice to look however you want is personal.

From a marketing standpoint, though, we have to be aware that every product featuring a Black woman on the box may not work for every Black woman. We can't always think, *She is Black, and this product must be for me.* We have been brainwashed. We have to remember that Black people come from families of multiple hair textures, so everything that is marketed to us may not work for me or for my sister. The heightened awareness of natural hair is definitely a movement, and it is not a fashion statement. I don't believe that it is a trend. I think that coming into who you are is a developmental process. I think the beginning of the hair and beauty journey is about freedom and self-expression.

Having been the parent of two tweens, I find that age group is really interesting, because most choose to socialize based on music. I think that many young girls who are eight to twelve years old can't wait to relax their hair because their icons all have smooth hair. If all of their music icons wear their hair straight, then that's the image that young girls will want for themselves. I think that, as the women who wear natural hair are younger and appeal to that population, there will be a shift in young girls' interpretation of beauty. Natural hair will look and feel more familiar to them. I think that there's an evolution to this process for young women. As they become a little older, their icons may not be as trendy. As their personal icons change, I think they also evolve.

For adults, though, the decision to wear hair natural or processed can be based on convenience. Going natural means that when you decide to get up and look fabulous for an event, meeting, or presentation, you don't have to worry about your hair looking crazy when you arrive.

When I'm around women who embrace their natural hair, I notice that something happens. When I'm in the room at natural hair events, these women are celebrating who they are. They're saying by their actions, "We don't all have curly, wavy, or tight hair, but we all have hair, and it's all different kinds of hair." This is just refreshing to watch. I feel like I'm looking at people who have found their tribes.

This way of thinking about hair is unfamiliar to a lot of adults. This mindset, though, can change, and the process can get easier over time. For example, most of us say we can't drink as much water in the amounts we should when we exercise. But when you start exercising and sweating, believe me, you will drink water. You'll also drink fewer sweetened drinks. This change happens because of the whole physical experience. The same transition applies when it comes to wearing our hair natural. The first time you decide to wear your hair natural, go to work, and see that it's a rainy day, your reaction is different. You don't respond like you did when you used a chemical. Now you can say, "Oh. It's raining," and not have a different reaction. Your experience has changed your response, and your change also affected your reaction.

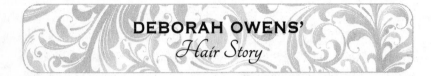

DEBORAH OWENS'
Hair Story

DEBORAH OWENS *is a sought-after financial expert and former financial executive whose mission is to help people build wealth. The CNN contributor can also be seen nationally on TVOne's* News One Now *program as "America's Wealth Coach." Deborah's weekly TVOne "WealthyU" segments help viewers navigate complexities of the economic landscape. Her ten-year stint as host of the NPR-affiliated* Wealthy Radio *broadcast has also created another platform for helping audiences develop a wealthy mindset at any income level. She often keynotes and provides corporate coaching to full audiences. Her acclaimed training sessions are founded on The Seven Wealthy Habits™ framework. Deborah's proprietary principles outline the attitudes, beliefs, and behaviors that help the masses take ownership of their personal, professional, and financial success. Deborah is also an author and wrote* Nickel and Dime Your Way to Wealth *and* A Purse of Your Own *(Simon & Schuster).*

When I started getting my hair braided, I was sort of stressed about being in an environment dominated by Caucasian males. I was the vice president, and I was very uncomfortable with how I would be perceived. I can remember that after I left a company, I was having a business meeting with someone who was going to be a potential client. She was an African-American, and I could just tell she was judging me. I really feel like her judgment of me was that I was not savvy enough to know what it took to make it in the business world. That meeting went nowhere.

I think how others perceive you has a lot to do with the choices you make. Women put in tremendous effort to look a certain way. Most women look the part and have the purses but have no money in their purses because it is expensive to maintain that. Think about it; even if you had invested $100 dollars a month in Apple stock, in ten years, it would be worth $142,000 dollars. That's my whole thing; people say, "Oh, I don't have the money." But yes, you do.

Natural hair and locs are not inexpensive, either. I have a friend who has to have her hair done every two weeks, and I think she pays $80 or $90 to have them twisted. I have been in a hair salon that is multicultural, and I have seen women who come in and want to be blond. They have to have their roots done. For some reason, if we have short hair, we want long, and if we have long, we want short. The fact is that the perceptions that women have about their looks cost a fortune at every level.

Not only Black women but all women need to begin to make some choices about how the decisions they are making today might impact them. When we talk about hair, we are talking about something that is going to impact us in the short term. The shift in our thinking really determines where we will go as women. Poor women think day to day. Working people think week to week. Middle class people think month to month, and rich people think year to year. Now, wealthy people think differently; wealthy people think decade to decade. It is so critical for women to think about a long-range plan.

We can't change what we will not acknowledge. It is important to begin to think about how hair is driving some of the financial decisions that we make. Some of these decisions may not be made in our own best interests. Think about the decisions that you are making today and how they are going to impact you in the long run.

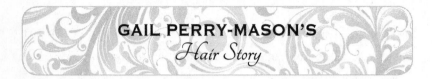

GAIL PERRY-MASON'S
Hair Story

GAIL PERRY-MASON *is a respected authority in the financial industry. The co-author of the bestselling* Girl, Make Your Money Grow! *(Random House) also founded Money Matters for Youth. Based in Detroit Public Schools, Gail teaches financial literacy and outlines the steps to entrepreneurship through this program. In 2014, Warren Buffett chose Money Matters for Youth as one of two organizations to donate the proceeds from the sales of Warren Buffet Fatheads. She regularly addresses full crowds to educate them on financial literacy and has conducted financial training sessions and workshops for companies such as Chrysler, IBM, MGM, McDonald's, DTE Energy, Blue Cross Blue Shield of Michigan, and Wells Fargo. Gail has been featured in many publications, including* Ebony, Black Enterprise, On Wall Street, CNN Money, Essence, *and* Associated Press. *Gail is also a mother of three terrific sons.*

I was adopted when I was three years old. I was labeled "special needs," and it was said that I would never be able to walk or talk. I was eventually adopted into an African-American family. My biological mother was White, and my biological father was Black. My hair is actually more like his hair than my mother's hair.

My mother gave me up because of what I looked like. She didn't even want to look at me or touch me because I was African-American. I met her a while ago, and she said to me, "You know I could have never done your hair. You would have just been bald-headed." I think when we adopt children with a different hair texture than ours, it is a learning process. We have to take special care and consideration of their hair, just like we do with everything else that relates to them. I see some people who adopt or people who have biracial kids. I've seen the way that they take care of the kid's hair; they just cut it all off into a little Afro. This will hurt their self-esteem in the long run.

My heart goes out to these children. Some things, you can cross over. You can cross over music. You can cross over everything else, but you can't cross over hair products. It's just like experts in finance or medicine can't switch specialties; it's the same exact thing. You cannot put a kiddie perm on a baby from China. You can damage a child's hair and make it all fall out.

Growing up, I had some friends who had hair that never frizzed up. I wanted a Kiddie Kit Relaxer, and would always think, *Why can't have I hair like theirs?* Now, I am so happy that I have thick, coarse hair. I now know that hair connects with emotions and says a lot about you. While I think hair is your crown, I don't think it makes you who you are. I think that back in the day, growing up, guys always looked at hair. Especially in the African-American community, they looked at the color and length. I know that some guys only dated girls depending on their hair and their skin color. While this is ridiculous to me, their idea of beauty definitely affected some women's self-esteem.

All women are princesses, and they all have a crown, no matter what type of hair they have. I think it's special, and it's something that God gave you. We should take care of our hair just like we take care of our bodies and everything else that God has given us.

Combing Through Chapter 7, The Split Ends

What part of the H.A.I.R. acronym most relates to you? Why?

_____

_____

What practical steps can you take to put these tips into practice?

_____

_____

Sometimes, partnerships accelerate the healing process. What connection can you make to help you move toward being whole? How can you connect with someone else and move them along in their process of self-acceptance?

_____

_____

Fill in this blank: I would love to feel more connected to myself as it relates to my _____

_____

What can you do to mend the split between who you are now and who you want to become?

_____

_____

Jot down some kind words—or *hairlooms*—about your hair.

_____

_____

Challenge yourself to compliment someone else using your own kind hair words!

_____

_____

Diagram Your "Mane" Issue

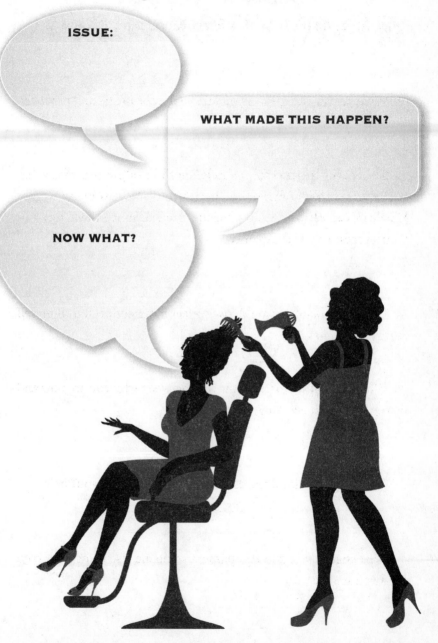

New Growth: Chart Your Solution		
Now What?	What's the Effect?	What's Your Solution?

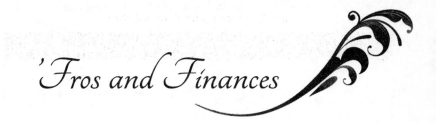

'Fros and Finances

How can we *mane*tain great-looking hair and stay afloat financially? *Hairlooms* financial experts have some tips to keep our hair and finances "on fleek":

Gail Perry Mason

- ◆ Decide which hair care regimens you really need versus the hair cares services that aren't essential.
- ◆ Cash in your clothes for a hairdo. Consider taking your clothes to a consignment shop and using the money from selling the items for a hairdo.

Cheryl Broussard

- ◆ Live in the present. Stop following people who are not in your income bracket. Until you get to the point where they are financially, stop trying to live like them.
- ◆ Position yourself to make more money. If you want to be able to afford these luxuries, such as hairstyles, you have to bring in more money.

- Use your talents to create a side business. Keep your nine-to-five, but don't have it as your only source of income. You should have three or four other ways to build your assets.

Deborah Owens

- The first thing you have to do is have a wealth system. Initially, put away whatever amount of money you feel like you can afford. This will point you in the right direction about what to do with your hair.
- Make a commitment to be able to do your hair yourself.
- Make sure you have a style you can maintain.
- Ask and answer this question for yourself—*How is what I'm doing today going to impact me in the long run?* If you just ask yourself that one question, you will make different decisions about your hair spending habits.

Hairlooms Strand Strategies

What's your natural hair and beauty goal? Maybe you want healthier hair or a better image of yourself in your own eyes. Have you reached it? Whether you've hit the mark or keep missing it, strategies will help us reach our destinations over time. Below are some practical steps I have taken and continue to take along my journey. These strategies are easy enough for you to implement, so let's get started!

#1: Bed? Head!

Depending on when you read this strategy, some of you may be heading to bed in a few hours. We all prepare for a good night's sleep in several ways. A warm cup of herbal tea or a dimly lit room is just what you may need to slip into the land of dreams.

Just what does it take to make sure your strands have a great night's sleep? Since I started being natural, I've realized that taking care great of my tresses at bedtime is so important. When I do, my hair shines as brightly as the next day's sun. Want to know what to consider? Here's what I've learned:

213

THREAD COUNTS: Some people fall asleep by counting sheep. If you're truly concerned about your hair, consider counting the threads in your sheets. Right after college, I had no clue about the importance of thread count. My bottom line was price. As a result, I slept on bedding that was stiff as a board and felt like paper. My pockets were happy, but my hair was hurting. In a few weeks, I noticed that the rough texture really made my hair dry. You may not be able to afford 1,200 thread count Egyptian cotton sheets, but consider affordable sheets with a thread count that won't sap your hair's moisture.

PILLOW TALK: Okay, okay. I know that great sheets can cost a small fortune. If you're cash-strapped, why not consider a satin pillow case? As I've transitioned with the quality of sheets, I've noticed that this pillow case has done the trick. Easy-breezy is the name of the game if you take this approach at night. I will typically prepare my hair for the next day and simply go to sleep. The satin pillow case keeps my hair from losing moisture or getting snagged in the pillow fabric.

IT'S A WRAP: When all else fails, the tried-and-true head scarf is also a great way to put your head to bed. After your nighttime "do" is in place, simply wrap it up and secure the scarf in the front or back of your head. Make sure, though, that you don't pick a scarf that will rob your hair of moisture. Consider scarves made from silky fabrics.

⊂✇⊃

#2: Three Tips for Manetaining Your Natural Hair

Have you ever wondered what to do with your natural 'do? There are days when it seems like chemically processed hair is the path of least resistance. As opposed to longing for the old, I've taken some time to simply understand how to deal with the *new*. Handling new growth at the time of a touch-up is one thing, but knowing how to handle a head of entirely natural hair can be a feat in itself. Whether you're wearing braids, a teeny-weeny Afro, or two-strand twists, consider these tips:

STAY ON "EDGE": For naturalistas, the edges of our hair are very delicate and least able to withstand the rigors of typical styling rituals. Excessive pulling will, over time, leave us with receding edges and a compromised hairline. I admit that there were times when I slathered my edges with heavy gels and pomades. I thought "laying my edges down" would give me the consummate, polished look. My hair may have looked good in the moment, but the build-up was hard to rinse from my hair without a lot of tugging. I'm currently resorting to kinder, gentler treatment of my edges. I make certain that they are neat, but not slick. After all, I'm a curly girl, and my edges weren't naturally designed to be straight!

"PIN IT" TO WIN IT: The winner in a wrestling match is always the individual who can pin the competitor. The victor has maneuvered in such a way that his partner's arms and legs are no longer moving, but subdued. Flyaway strands, twists, and curls have a way of taking over the perfect hairstyle. I have found that bobby pins are a great way to emerge picture perfect. Given the density and texture of my hair, I am able to use several at a time, and they rarely slip out of place. The neat thing about these must-haves is that they are dirt cheap. You can pay only pennies for enough clips—from your local beauty supply store—to last for a few months or a year.

JOIN THE "BAND": What would I do without headbands? Thank God I'll never have to know, because I keep a stash of them handy at all times. These plastic and fabric bands have the super power to change my look from dull to dynamite in a matter of seconds by adding a pop of color or a little bling to complement or liven up my outfit! Headbands can do double duty, not only adding style, but also repairing a problem. For example, at times, my two-strand twists start to unravel, or my twist-outs have seen better days. A headband is also a quick fix to keep my flyaway hairs neatly tucked when making a bun.

ᏧᏋᏅ

#3: Three 'Dos for "Natural Newbies"

Sometimes we just need to know what to do . . . with our 'do! For the past six years, I've found some tried-and-true 'dos that have taken me from the classroom to the boardroom in style. I know that a lot of natural women sport some more elaborate styles, but I tend to go for a simple look that I can manage on my own. As I keep exploring the wonders of my kinky curls, I'm sure I'll branch out. For now, though, enjoy my three 'fro faves:

Do #1—Two-Strand Twists: A lot of us may remember wearing this style as little girls. The two-strand twist, for me, was an alternative to the everyday braids my mother made me wear. This style can still work for us now that we're all grown up. Whether my hair was a few inches long or shoulder length, the process of simply sectioning my hair and twisting two strands around each other was pretty easy. Don't get me wrong—the first time I tried was a disaster, but with lots of practice, I eventually nailed the process.

Do #2—Roller-Set Twists: It's not uncommon to see women and girls wear twists that are not curled. I like to spice it up and roll up my twists for a completely different look. Try using smaller rollers for tighter curls and larger rollers for looser curls. Remember to always use rollers that are not too hard; your head will thank you in the morning. For the best roller twists, I sit under a dryer—either a soft bonnet dryer or a hard-top dryer for about thirty to forty minutes—set at a comfortable setting. Keep in mind, though, that your dryer time will vary based on your hair thickness and length. This technique gives my twists bounce that lasts for at least a couple of weeks.

Do #3—Twist-Out: I absolutely love this look. It's the easiest of the three. After a couple of weeks, I'll simply unwind my roller-set twists. I do this by gently unraveling each twist from the end until I reach the root are. This technique gives me an entirely new look. Depending on how wavy I want my hair, I can get about two to three days out of this style. After your twist-out is worn out, just wash and start styling again.

#4: Three Tips for Travelling Tresses

How do you handle your hair when you're not at home? We all have a personal regimen to make our hair perk up when we wake up. For those of us who are on the road, our "'do duty" can become a hassle. Stores may not carry our products, water may be harsh, and the TSA may confiscate our products before we ever land! These and other variables can make it tough to know whether our hair will be ready for the big reveal when we're miles away from home.

Worry not; I've traveled from Thailand to Texas since my hair has been natural. The experience has been a "trip" (pun intended), and I'm happy to offer you the benefit of my road-tested knowledge! These tips may help you maintain great-looking locks during your layovers:

"EYE" SPY: Who moves into a new neighborhood without researching clothing stores, schools, or malls? No one! So why would we travel without researching which stores carry our hair products? Make sure that *before you go Greyhound, go Google*. Find out where you can purchase your must-have products. You may deplete your travel stash—or may even forget to pack your product—and need to know where to get a new supply.

NEVER LAND: Much like Peter Pan, the mythical boy who lives in a land where he never grows up, we may say we'll never need our hair-care accessories. I've often said, "I'll *never* use those pins," or "I'll *never* use those combs," or "I'll *never* use those ponytail holders." Guess what? Everything I've said I'd never need, I needed. When packing, resist the urge to purge. Always carry extra pins, combs, and other hair accessories. The hair tool you leave at home could be the very thing you need to stay on top of your hair game while on the road.

"CAP" SIZE: A capsized canoe or kayak can turn a day on the water into a soggy mess. Likewise, a too-small shower cap can spell doom for your do. While most hotels offer shower caps, I've noticed that they're not sized to cover all of my natural hair. As a result, water gets under my cap, and my 'do is done! If you're on the go, always bring your own shower cap. This is the best way to make sure that your hair won't get wet when your body does!

ھ

#5: "Hair" Today ... Gone Tomorrow

Years ago, lots of my friends were getting extensions. I didn't want to be left out, so I joined in. I got some extensions for an event and wore them to that function. I loved being able to swing my hair. I loved having hair hang down my back. What I didn't love, though, was having my hair break off after wearing the tracks for just one week.

Based on my personal experience, I realize that hair health is linked to knowing how to: a) avoid hair loss, and b) stop hair loss before it starts. If your hair is thinning due to poor treatment or medicine, these tips will be helpful. If your hair is full, bouncing, and behaving, congratulations! Either way, the health of your hair is in your hands. You can be the boss! Consider these hair tips using the acronym BOSS:

BALANCE: What woman is not engaged in a daily juggling act? Finding time to bag lunches while cooking dinner and nailing business deals is no small feat. Every "ball" of responsibility is suspended midair, and you're doing everything to make sure nothing hits the floor! With the attention needed to execute all of these tasks—at times simultaneously—how can you carve out moments in a day for wrapping, braiding, or tying up hair at night? The key is balance. Plot out the amount of time needed for your hair routine and begin to weave other tasks in and out of this time frame. You may find that your balance comes by preplanning hair routines or selecting low-maintenance styles on super busy days. Balance will ensure that your hair doesn't get the short end of the priority stick!

OBSESSION: When it comes to hair, we have to know what 'do's are don'ts for us! Dyes, weaves, or perms may be great for a colleague but perhaps not for you. Don't become fixated on a look. Perhaps the best hair-care regimen should start with knowing what works best for you versus another woman.

SPEED: Rushing on the highway can get us a ticket. Likewise, speeding through our beauty regimen could mean we pay with our hair. Take time to see how your hair responds to certain treatments, products, or styles. If something's not working, slow down and consider making the *right turn* so your tresses aren't left on the roadside.

STRESS: Stress can take a toll on our skin, emotions, and—yes—our hair. Relational upheavals or ongoing financial challenges may be a recipe for hair loss. When possible, keep tabs on how you're doing spiritually, physically, and emotionally. If you're running on E (empty) on any of these tanks, do what's necessary to bring balance into your life.

∽

#6: Five Ways to Beat the Heat!

Heat damage wasn't an issue until I decided to wear my natural hair. Now that I've been a naturalista for more than seven years, this is a *hot topic* of discussion, because I want healthy hair. Knowing the amount of heat to use on your hair is the difference between fallout and growth. Whether you're transitioning, learning to rock your kinky coils, or a seasoned natural hair vet, these tips will be helpful:

TIP #1—KNOW THE SIGNS: Over time, I realized that no amount of washing and conditioning could rid my hair of a distinctive smell: burnt hair! Even though my hair had been flat-ironed months ago, the burnt hair smell lingered. As if that wasn't bad enough, then I noticed more-than-normal shedding.

TIP #2—CHECK THE TEMPERATURE: As a girl, I remember sneaking to hot comb my hair. I should have known danger was lurking when I lifted the hot comb from the fire and part of it was white! White-hot coals are great for the grill but spell D-I-S-A-S-T-E-R for natural hair. Hot combs, curling irons, and flat irons should be no hotter than 375 degrees Fahrenheit.

TIP #3—MIX IT UP: After my hair suffered heat damage, I didn't know what I was going to do. I was so used to achieving straight hair with direct heat. Over time, I learned that air drying and bonnet dryers are great alternatives. Depending on how I prep my hair, I can still pull off a great look with less direct heat.

TIP #4—CUT IT OFF: You couldn't have told me seven years ago that I'd be so excited about a haircut. After this last round of heat damage, I almost begged my stylist to cut it off. Five months later, I'm so glad I did. Sometimes trimming or starting over is the best way to handle heat damage because you know you're starting with a clean slate.

TIP #5—LOVE YOURSELF: I saved the hardest tip for last. The first time I cut my hair because of heat damage, I really struggled with feeling ugly. I believed the lie that long hair—regardless of its condition—made me pretty and valuable. The second time around, though, I had worked through enough issues to know that I am beautiful inside and out. My hair doesn't make me; God made me. That fact alone means I'm a beauty, and you are too!

&⌖9

#7: Tips for Transitioning to Natural Hair Without Losing Your Mind

For many Black women, their first chemical relaxer is a rite of passage! Getting a perm every four to six weeks seamlessly ushers Black women into the ranks of other Aunties, Big Mamas, Nanas, and Sista-Friends who have undergone this beauty treatment for decades.

Data findings project that Black women in the United States are expected to spend a whopping $72 million on perms.[1] Nonetheless, many are breaking ranks! If you plan to make the switch, consider these tips before you transition:

UNDERSTAND YOUR "WHY": In a lot of instances, transitions don't come without opposition. I've already talked about the inner and outer struggles of going against society's beauty grain. The only thing that made me persevere was my rock-solid conviction. I stopped perming for two reasons: a) I didn't want perm-related chemicals in my bloodstream while carrying a baby, and b) I was tired of throwing money away on perms that couldn't hold up under perspiration or a few raindrops. Do you *really* know why you want to transition? Why is it important to have your roots show and fuzzy edges? When you—for yourself—clearly understand why you're changing, the transition will be smooth.

KNOW THE PRICE: Ancient wisdom in the Bible states that it's best to count the cost of a project before jumping in![2] So it is with a transition from a perm to natural hair. There are literal costs associated with ditching a perm that are often overlooked. With my accumulation of trial-and-error natural hair care products, I could have operated a modest natural hair care section from the comfort of my bathroom. You may spend $50 trying to find the right sulfate-free shampoo, and someone else may fork over $250 when searching for the best co-wash. While your expenses will vary, remember that the transition needed to properly care for your natural tresses isn't free—there is a cost!

EXPECT TO LOOK DIFFERENT: I can hear a chorus of *"Duh"* after reading the title of this tip! While this thought is a no-brainer, I really was expecting my natural hair to respond like my permed hair. After using tons of gel and water combos, it finally sunk in that my natural hair is wavier, kinkier, and curlier than I knew. Not only that, but I had to accept that my physical appearance had shifted. Don't fool yourself like I did and believe that your hair will look the same. I was able to cross this hurdle by constantly reminding myself that looking different is not bad; it's just different. As you step into the beginning hours, days, and weeks without a perm, just remember that your wave pattern is not bad. Your wave pattern is different, and different is still beautiful!

⊰⊱

#8: Does Your Style "Work Out"?

Making the decision to go natural definitely presented a new set of challenges when I hit the gym at work. Maybe you started working out before you hit the office—like I did—and eventually started exercising during your work day. Is it possible to have an on-the-job fitness routine and still keep your hair intact? With a little flexibility and a lot of planning, you and your 'fro can get fit at work! Here's how:

WORK AFTER HOURS: The time to try new hairdos is not when you're scrambling to get to work on time. The time to try new styling options for your post-workout hair is after hours. For example, try a new style after a weekend workout. Getting creative on a Saturday or Sunday will really help you explore new looks without the pressure of having to be ready immediately. Using your off days is also a great time to get feedback from those closest to you about the styles that best suit your authentic self!

CHECK YOUR TIME: If you apply the previous tip, no doubt you'll have at least a few new styles under your belt. The next phase is to consider the amount of time it takes for each style against your work schedule. For example, on deadline days, I knew I had to pick a style that I could whip into shape with no problems. Fridays were slower paced for me in the office; on those days, I could select a style that took longer to perfect. Why? Because I scheduled my 'do around my day! Consider timing your hair prep, and make the necessary adjustments based on your professional responsibilities.

ALWAYS BE PREPARED: I can't tell you how many times I left the office gym with sopping wet curls. Over time, I wasn't on high alert because I learned to stash bobby pins, pony-tail holders, and other hair accessories in my purse. When packing your gym clothes, towel, and toiletries, don't forget your hair care "rescue kit." You may want to get a separate travel-size case that's used for trial size products and/or hair tools that keep your hair on point regardless of the intensity of your workout.

⚬⚮⚬

#9: How to Detangle with Ease!

I already know that most of us grimace when we think of detangling. Knots and snarls have somehow crept into our luscious locks, and we need to deal with them before they get worse. Perhaps you didn't wear a protective wrap at night, and now your hair is matted. Maybe you made your two-strand twists too tiny—this is me—and now you're paying the price with hair that's tangled. Your hair may be in knots, but there is a way out! Here's what I've learned along the way:

DITCH YOUR EMOTIONS: I remember wearing braids as a preteen. They were cute going in, but taking them out was another story. After an hour of wrestle mania, I got out my scissors, and the rest was history. Looking back, I realize my choice to cut was based on my frustration and not the tangles. Ladies, please don't let your feelings get the best of you when doing your hair. If you're agitated because your hair is breaking, not laying straight, or not looking like that magazine picture, step away and come back when you're calm. In my case, I charged ahead and cut my braids in a fit of rage; in the next moment, I was looking at a bald patch that lasted for months. Detangling during heated moments may give us a quick fix but create permanent hair problems!

HANDLE WITH CARE: Rough-and-tumble is great for footballs, but not for our hair! When my precious niece was born the whole family gently reminded my rambunctious nephew to be "soft and gentle." His tendency was to pounce and pull, and so is some of ours! Contrary to appearance and popular belief, our hair is fragile and has to be handled gently. Start detangling at the ends and slowly work your way toward the roots. If you get frustrated, give yourself a break and come back to the process when you're more calm.

CHOOSE YOUR TOOLS: When it comes to detangling natural hair, one way doesn't always work. When my hair was shoulder length, my go-to tactic was a wide tooth comb and a Denman-type brush. Now that I'm sporting a short Afro, my hair actually does best when I finger comb it. Pay attention to how your hair responds during each natural hairstyle you choose. What works best when unraveling Bantu knots? How do you deal with matted two-strand twists? As you analyze your hair's response to being handled, it will be clear which method to use.

◌✑◌

#10: *How to Make and Break Your Hair Journey Resolutions*

We've all been there. Our seasonal hair promises can be endless. January may look great, but June can look like a mess! Consider why we may have missed it in the past. It's as simple as A-B-C:

A—WE AIM TOO HIGH: You know we can bite off more than we can chew. Certain statements—*we'll always trim our ends on time* or *we'll never use harsh chemicals*—set us up to fail.
Solution: Pick one small, achievable goal. Conquer it, and celebrate your victory. Over time, small successes will equal total success!

B—WE BELIEVE WE CAN'T: If you believe you can't, you won't. Whatever we plan to do with our hair is based on our actions. No hair stylist or loctician is going to make us "do our 'do"!

Solution: Remind yourself of what you've done in the past. "Comb through" your life and see where you hit the mark. If you did it before, you can do it again in another area of your life!

True story: in 2015, I kept saying, "I can't cornrow my hair." After these negative thoughts, I realized that these "same hands" that crochet can cornrow! Over time, I learned to do it despite my initial negative words.

C—WE CHOOSE TO COMPARE: I know I sound like a broken record, but *don't compare your hair!* You may hit your hair goal in August, and someone else will reach it in April. That makes sense because everyone's hair is different and responds differently.

Solution: Get to know the hair on your head. When you know what you've got, make hair resolutions that are sensible. Eventually you'll see great results for *your* hair, and the change won't be based on someone else's.

Basic Steps
for Healthy Hair

by *Hairlooms* contributor Karen Wilson, of Karen Wilson Beauty

Healthy Hair Tips for Women with Wavy/Curly Hair

Wavy and curly hair is naturally drier than straight hair textures. So you need to allow your hair's sebum (i.e., natural oily secretions) to lubricate your hair shaft.

- ◆ Gently massage your scalp to increase blood circulation.
- ◆ Cleanse your hair using a sulfate-free shampoo no more than once per week. Always follow each shampoo with a conditioner. Detangle hair by fingering and/or combing through hair while the conditioner is in.
- ◆ Use a high-quality, deep-penetrating conditioner for an intense treatment at least once per month. Cover using a plastic cap and sit under a hooded dryer for at least twenty minutes.

◆ First, use fingers to detangle your hair. If necessary, follow up using a wide-tooth comb and gently detangle your hair.

◆ Always use a leave-in conditioner after rinsing out your conditioner. This helps to detangle your hair and closes your cuticle layer of hair.

◆ Pay close attention to moisturizing your ends, as they are usually the driest part of your hair.

◆ Get your ends trimmed at least four times per year. If you do not trim your ends, they will continue to split further up your hair shaft. If you frequently style your hair, get your ends trimmed every two to three months.

◆ Minimize the use of heat appliances on your hair (e.g., flat irons, curling irons). Too much heat will cause dry, brittle hair, and may also lead to hair loss. Use a thermal protector or serum on your hair to protect it from the heat when using heat appliances.

◆ Use hair products that contain or are derived from natural ingredients, as these products do not strip your hair of its natural essential oils and nutrients.

◆ Stay away from products containing rubbing alcohol, sulphate, mineral oil, petroleum, astringents, chemicals, and other synthetic ingredients. These harsh ingredients will cause dry, brittle hair if used over an extended period of time, and they may not be easily absorbed by the hair shaft.

Healthy Hair Tips for Women with Straight Hair

◆ Comb or brush your dry hair before washing it to break up and remove excess dirt. Never use a brush on wet hair, which may lead to hair breakage.

- Cleanse your hair using a natural and sulfate-free shampoo as often as needed. The frequency of shampooing will be based on how dry and oily your hair is. Natural shampoos will not strip your hair of its essential oils and nutrients. Follow each shampoo with a conditioner. Use cool water to rinse and help seal in the moisture as the cuticle closes.

- Deep conditioning is essential to maintaining healthy hair. Deep condition hair at least once per week to improve the overall look and feel of your hair.

- Gently squeeze your hair to release excess water, and then blot it with a towel.

- Brush hair when it is dry, but avoid using plastic hairbrushes.

- Minimize the use of heat appliances on your hair (e.g., flat iron, curling iron). Too much heat will cause dry, brittle hair, and may also lead to hair loss. Use a thermal protector or serum on your hair to protect it from the heat when using heat appliances, set your styling tools on a low setting, and never use hair straighteners on wet hair.

- Let your hair air dry naturally to prevent damage from a hairdryer. If you need to use a hairdryer, let your hair air dry as much as possible before using it.

- Get your ends trimmed at least four times per year. If you do not trim your ends, they will continue to split further up your hair shaft.

- A healthy lifestyle affects healthy hair! Drink plenty of water, eat proper foods, and exercise!

Hairstyles and Styling Tips for Children with Wavy/Curly Hair

◆ **Ponytails.** Ponytails are always an easy and age-appropriate style for children. Keep in mind that wavy/curly hair is not straight, so don't pull the ponytail so tight where it places tension on your hairline—this may lead to hair loss. Use hair balls, coated elastic bands, or nylon- or satin-covered rubber bands to protect against breakage. Remove bands at night and braid hair into small sections to cut back on detangling.

◆ **Wash-'n'-Go.** This style is as simple as it gets! Make sure hair is clean and tangle-free. While hair is saturated with water, apply a curling cream, natural gel, or leave-in conditioner on small to medium sections of the hair to define natural curls. Allow hair to air dry or have the child sit under a hooded dryer that is placed on low to medium heat for about thirty minutes (dryer time is contingent upon length and density of hair). To maintain control of voluminous hair and to accessorize this look, use a headband! Make sure the band is not rubber and does not have small teeth on the inside of the band, which will tear the hair.

◆ **Two-Strand Twists.** Twists are an attractive style for children. This style is achieved by taking two sections of hair (about half an inch each) and crossing one section of hair over the other section to create a two-strand twist. To spice it up, place a colorful flower in the front of her hair after it dries, or secure twists with decorative barrettes and clips. For bedtime maintenance, cover the hair with a silk scarf or satin bonnet. Note: the coarser the hair texture, the better the twist will hold. Finer-textured hair may require the use of rubber bands to secure the twists.

◆ **Two-Strand Twist-Out.** A variation on the two-strand twist hairstyle is a two-strand twist-out. After the twists have fully dried, take each twist and separate it into two twists. For a fuller effect, separate into three or four sections. You may adorn this style by placing a headband further back on top of the head to help control the direction of the hair. Bedtime maintenance may require the hair to be retwisted in larger sections to help maintain curl pattern and reduce tangling.

◆ **Braids.** Braided hair can look artistic, creative, and very attractive on children. Braids also allow children to engage in playtime and activities without hair falling in their faces. Add colored beads at the ends of the braids to complement the child's attire. In order to maintain moisture, mist braided hair with water, conditioning spray, or oil. To alleviate a dry and itchy scalp, oil the scalp about twice per week, or as needed. It is important to use natural oil such as tea tree or jojoba—not "grease" or petroleum-based oils. Braids can be left in for about four to six weeks.

Be sure hair is braided gently at the hairline. Braiding hair too tightly may cause traction alopecia, which is hair loss caused by excessively pulling or tugging the hair. Styles that are too tight can also lead to thinning and baldness. For bedtime maintenance, tie a silk scarf around the hair. Braids are recommended for children with relaxed hair.

◆ **Roller and Rod Sets.** Redefine your child's natural curls by placing them on rollers and rods. The size of the rollers or rods will determine the size of the curls. Keep in mind that a loosely rolled curl will quickly frizz and lose shape. If your child tends to perspire a lot or struggles to keep her hair neat, tight curls may be the better choice.

Any of these styles can be combined to create a new style. Try a two-strand twist-out ponytail, or braid your child's hair from the hairline to the crown, leaving a curly 'fro in the back. Be as creative as you like!

Hairstyles and Styling Tips for Children with Straight Hair

- **Ponytails**. Ponytails are always an easy and age-appropriate style for children. Use nylon- or satin-covered rubber bands to protect against breakage. Remove bands at night.
- **Bangs**. Bangs are a quick and easy way to give straight hair style!
- **Curls**. Add curls to straight hair by setting the hair on hair rollers, or using a curling iron on a low setting. Create pin curls for bedtime maintenance. Give your child's curls a little more character by accessorizing this look with the addition of a colored headband! Make sure band is not rubber and does not have small teeth on the inside of the band, which will tear the hair.
- **French braids**. Braids are unique and fun. French braids and side braids are an easy and attractive way to style straight hair. As an alternative style, unbraid hair to give it a wavy texture and definition.

Hair and Beauty Resources

Jane Carter
www.janecartersolution.com

Gwen Jimmere
www.naturalicious.net

Lisa Price
www.carolsdaughter.com

Karen Wilson
karenwilsonnaturalbeauty.com

Diane Cole Stevens
www.colestevenssalon.com

The PuffCuff
www.thepuffcuff.com

Ceata E. Lash is the founder and inventor of the PuffCuff, which is the only hair clamp designed for thick, curly, textured hair. Launched in 2014, this hair clamp has emerged as a new hair accessory designed to solve the woes of women frustrated with seeking a way to gather their curls into a ponytail or updo. The PuffCuff is designed with lightweight, impact-resistant plastic that does not cause hair breakage or damage and works with all types of thick hair—including thick or wavy curls, locs, twists, and braids. All PuffCuffs are made in the USA.

Food and Fitness

Nicole Ari Parker
saveyourdo.com

Toni Carey
blackgirlsrun.com

Dr. Ro
www.everythingro.com

Vivian Joiner
www.sweetpotatoes.ws

Finances

Cheryl Broussard
www.cherylbroussard.com

Deborah Owens
www.deborahowens.com

Emotional Health and Wellness Resources

Melissa Gordon-Pitts, MSW, LCSW-C, LCSW, is the founder of Core Health Counseling. Core Health is a Concierge Mental Health Therapy Practice serving Northern Virginia, the District of Columbia, and the Baltimore metro areas. Onsite and web-based counseling services allow Core Health Counseling to provide high-quality, caring services worldwide.

Counseling areas include:

- Individual counseling
- Couples counseling
- Family counseling
- Premarital counseling

www.corehealthcounseling.com

Nichola Brown, MSW, LICSW, is a Licensed Independent Clinical Social Worker in private practice with professional experience across a wide range of areas. Her specialty areas are depression and anxiety, and her practice's core offerings also include wellness for individuals, stress management, and workplace stress and burnout recovery. Nichola's hope is that her clients find wholeness in the midst of their brokenness. Nichola is also the author of *Sabbath Season: A Call to Rest,* which is a resource to complement her approach to lifestyle wellness.

www.keilahrestoration.com

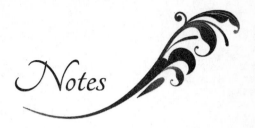

Notes

Introduction

1. Pentagon Does About-Face on Hair Regulations—Black Women Approve. National Public Radio, August 14, 2014. *http://www.npr.org/sections/codeswitch/2014/08/13/340155211/pentagon -does-about-face-on-hair-regulations-black-women-approve*

2. Female Marines in Uniform Can Now Wear Locks and Twists in Their Hair. *Stars and Stripes*, December 15, 2015. *http://www.stripes.com/news/female-marines-in-uniform-can-now-wear -locks-and-twists-in-their-hair-1.384225*

3. Tamron Hall Wears Her Natural Hair for the First Time on TV. *TODAY*, June 27, 2014. *http:// www.today.com/style/tamron-hall-wears-her-natural-hair-first-time-tv-t73346*

4. Hair-Bullying and the Decline of U.S. Education System. *The Huffington Post*, June 2, 2014. *http://www.huffingtonpost.com/ama-yawson/hairbullying-and-the-decl_b_5068354.html*

5. Sheryl Underwood Black Hair Comments Apology. *Steve Harvey Show* audio file. *https://www. youtube.com/watch?v=PDqo-NqFEPM*

6. Katie Couric Wigs Out on Hair-Themed "Katie" Today—SNEAK PEEK. *Entertainment Weekly*, September 19, 2012. *http://www.ew.com/article/2012/09/19/katie-couric-hair-show*

7. LaFrance, M. (2001). First Impressions and Hair Impressions: An Investigation of Impact of Hairstyle on First Impressions. Unpublished manuscript. Department of Psychology, Yale University, New Haven, CT.

Chapter 1: Baby Hairs

1. Beauty by the Numbers. The Benchmarking Company, March 2016. *http://www.benchmark ingcompany.com*

2. *http://wwd.com/beauty-industry-news/color-cosmetics/essence-panel-explores-beauty-pur chasing-2139829/* "Essence Beauty Panel Explores Beauty Purchasing"

3. Gabby Douglas's Hair Sets Off Twitter Debate, but Some Ask: "What's the Fuss?" *The Washington Post*, August 3, 2012. *https://www.washingtonpost.com/lifestyle/style/gabby-douglass-hair-sets -off-twitter-debate-but-some-ask-whats-the-fuss/2012/08/03/38548064-ddaf-11e1-9ff9 -1dcd8858ad02_story.html*

Chapter 2: Check Your Roots

1. *Lift Ev'ry Voice and Sing.* Text: James Weldon Johnson (1871–1938), alt. and Tune: J. Rosamond Johnson (1873–1954), Copyright: Public Domain.

Chapter 3: Dread Locks

1. *Fear*, Michele Tapp © 1985.
2. *The Colored American*, Edward Elder Cooper: Washington, DC. 1893–1904. Copyright: Public Domain.

Chapter 4: The Mane Attraction

1. Why Women Talk More than Men: Language Protein Uncovered, *Science World Report*, February 20, 2013. *http://www.scienceworldreport.com/articles/5073/20130220/why-women-talk-more-men-language-protein.htm*
2. Doctors Kenneth and Mamie Clark and "The Doll Test." NAACP Legal Defense and Educational Fund, Inc. *http://www.naacpldf.org/brown-at-60-the-doll-test*

Chapter 5: Hair Peace

1. Holland, Stephanie. Marketing to Women Quick Facts: Women and Spending. *Sheconomy*. *http://she-conomy.com/report/marketing-to-women-quick-facts*
2. Surgeon General: Don't Let Hair Get in the Way. *National Public Radio News*, August 8, 2012. *http://www.npr.org/2012/08/08/158419580/surgeon-general-dont-let-hair-get-in-the-way*

Chapter 6: Pony Tales

1. Willie Lynch: *The Making of a Slave. www.bnpublishing.com*
2. *Born in Slavery: Slave Narratives from the Federal Writers' Project, 1936–1938*. Georgia Narratives: Volume IV, Part 2, Life Viewed by an Ex Slave, pp. 259–260, Manuscript Division, Library of Congress.
3. *Born in Slavery: Slave Narratives from the Federal Writers' Project, 1936-1938*. Georgia Narratives: Volume IV, Part 4, Life Viewed by an Ex Slave, pp. 35–36, Manuscript Division, Library of Congress.
4. *Pony Tales*, Michele Tapp Roseman © 2016.
5. *Born in Slavery: Slave Narratives from the Federal Writers' Project, 1936–1938*. Georgia Narratives: Volume IV, Part 2, Life Viewed by an Ex Slave, pp. 259–260, Manuscript Division, Library of Congress.
6. Edmonia Lewis Biography. *Biography.com. http://www.biography.com/people/edmonia-lewis-9381053*
7. BlackPast.org. *http://www.blackpast.org/aah/reed-judy-w-c-1826*
8. *ExplorePAhistory.org. http://explorepahistory.com/hmarker.php?markerId=1-A-282*

Hairlooms Strand Strategies

1. "Natural Hair, Don't Care: Why More Black Women Are Avoiding Chemical Relaxers", TakePart Digital News and Lifestyle Magazine, April 19, 2015. *http://www.takepart.com/article/2015/04/19/chemical-hair*
2. Luke 14:28 (New International Version)

Color Yourself Beautiful!

Art therapists have long known that creating art is a great way to untangle emotional knots and begin the healing process. On the following page is an illustration that is just waiting for your unique, creative touches. There is no right or wrong way to color—just explore and have fun! As you shade in each area, reflect on the beautiful and unique ways that *you* color the world.

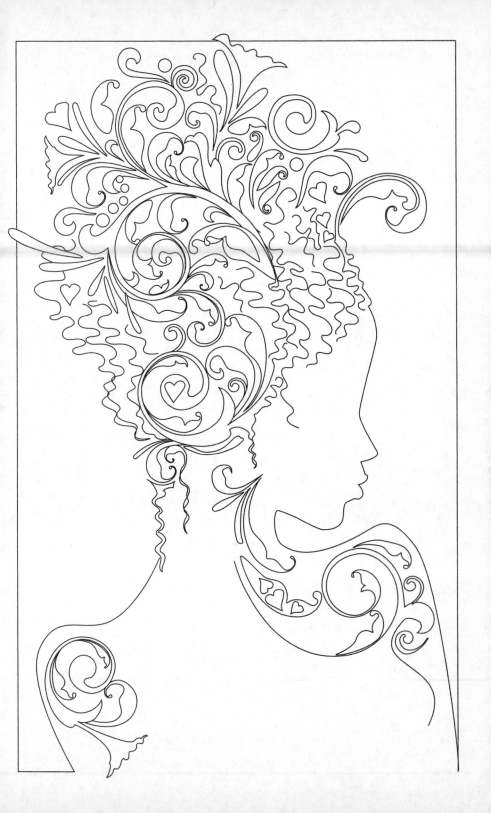

An Invitation from Michele

Thanks so much for joining me on the journey to develop an inside-out love. The pathway to self-acceptance is always easier when you're not walking alone. If you enjoyed the *Hairlooms* experience, let's keep the conversation flowing! Here's how:

1. Email me directly at *info@hairloomsthebook.com* to share your thoughts or just to say, "hi"!
2. Visit *hairloomsthebook.com* for helpful blog content, personal growth tips, contest/giveaway information, and *Hairlooms* experience updates.
3. Use the hashtag *#HairloomsTheBook* when posting your coloring page photos and comments on social media.
4. Leave a review on *amazon.com, barnesandnoble.com,* and *booksamillion.com.*

About the Author

Michele Tapp Roseman is a seasoned writer with contributions in print and electronic media, as well as a media placement specialist. She earned an MA in Journalism and Public Affairs from American University and a BA in English from Bucknell University.

Michele was the Senior Producer for Wealthy Radio, which broadcasts weekly on NPR-affiliated WEAA in Baltimore, Maryland. In this capacity she secured interviews with several high-profile individuals, including: Jim Cramer, CNBC's *Mad Money* host and author of *Get Rich Carefully*; Marc Ecko, billion-dollar Ecko brand founder and author of *Unlabel*; and Pat Neely, Food Network celebrity chef and co-author of *The Neelys' Celebration Cookbook*.

Michele has also attracted media coverage on behalf of President Barack Obama's Special Assistant for Disability Policy on WUSA-TV (CBS affiliate). As the personal publicist for Academy Award-winning actor Jeff Bridges, she secured significant press coverage in support of his role in Showtime's Emmy-nominated docudrama, "Hidden in America." For Elder Bernice King (Dr. Martin Luther King's daughter), Michele placed her on the nationally acclaimed *The Bible Experience* project.

As an editorial consultant, Michele has taught courses in Bangkok, Thailand, and trained foreign nationals from Afghanistan, Mozambique, Peru, and Taiwan. She has also provided consulting services within government agencies and on military bases throughout the United States. The native New Yorker is a songwriter and enjoys crocheting. She resides in Maryland with her husband, Kyle.

A Gallery of Hairlooms Contributors

On the following pages are photos of the esteemed individuals I was honored to personally interview for *Hairlooms*. Each graciously shared personal stories that touched on some aspect of self-acceptance for Black women. Their poignant accounts can illuminate the way for all of us as we the beauty that resides within.